HUNTINGTON'S DISEASE

The Best Science in Everyday Language

JERRY BELLER HEALTH RESEARCH INSTITUTE

DEDICATION

To people living with Dementia and their loved ones.

CONTENTS

FOREWORD 1

Who is the reading audience? 5

Two Dementia Series 14

I. DEMENTIA 16

Chapter 1: WHAT IS DEMENTIA? 17

Chapter 2: WHAT ARE THE 19 PRIMARY DEMENTIAS? 21

Chapter 3: WHO IS MOST LIKELY TO GET DEMENTIA? 24

Chapter 4: DEMENTIA COSTS & PREVALENCE 35

II. HUNTINGTON'S DISEASE 48

Chapter 5: WHAT IS HUNTINGTON'S DISEASE (HD)? 49

HUNTINGTON'S DISEASE SYMPTOMS & STAGES 56

Chapter 6: HUNTINGTON'S DISEASE SYMPTOMS 57

Chapter 7: HUNTINGTON'S DISEASE (HD)-RELATED SUICIDE 59

Chapter 8: HUNTINGTON'S STAGES 62

IV. HUNTINGTON'S DISEASE (HD) RISK FACTORS 73

Chapter 9: HUNTINGTON'S DISEASE CAUSE & RISK FACTORS 74

V. BONUS SECTION 76

Chapter 10: Starter To-do List for Somebody and Family once Diagnosed with Dementia. 77

Chapter 12: CARE TEAM 86

Chapter 13: LETTER TO CONGRESS 89

CONCLUSION..91

THANK YOU FOR READING 95

BELLER HEALTH BOOKS...96

Other Beller Health Books...99

ABOUT THE AUTHOR 100

ACKNOWLEDGMENTS

Thanks to the American Academy of Neurology, Atlanta Center for Medical Research, Alzheimer's Association, Alzheimer's Disease Center, Alzheimer's Disease Center of Northwestern University, Alzheimer's Foundation of America, American Academy of Neurology, Association for Frontotemporal Degeneration, Australia Neurological Research, CDC, Department of Health and Human Services, Duke University Medical Center, Emory Hospital, Harvard Medical School, Johns Hopkins Medicine, Mayo Clinic, National Aphasia Association, National Institute of Neurological Disorders and Strokes, National Library of Medicine, National Institute on Aging, National Institutes of Health, Prince of Wales Medical Research Institute, *PubMed*, Stanford Library School of Medicine, Stanford Medicine, UCSF Department of Neurology, UCSF Memory and Aging Center, University of Cambridge Neurology Unit, World Health Organization (WHO), *Journal of American Medical Association* (JAMA), and several other organizations that provided information used for this book. Thanks to everybody who assisted this book in a variety of important ways, and everybody at Beller Health Research Institute. To my editor, John Briggs, who helps me improve every book. To all sources and for the photos. Most of all, thanks to my wife, Nicola Beller

FOREWORD

Before diving into the book's subject matter, let's discuss two related Dementia series:

- *2020 Dementia Overview* series
- *2020 Dementia Types, Symptoms, Stages, & Risk Factors* series

2020 Dementia Overview series is an extension of the medical groundbreaking *19 Dementia Types, Symptoms, Stages, & Risk Factors* series, the first covering all primary dementia types.

After spending decades building an audience in other genres, including nutrition, circumstances turned the world upside down. Doctors diagnosed my mother with Alzheimer's. The same doctors soon diagnosed my father with cancer. A few months later, my father's favorite brother and my closest uncle died.

Three consecutive hard blows blew the world beyond recognition.

Tough and decent as they come, dad insisted on taking care of my mother while fighting brain cancer. My brothers and sister-in-law did their share, but Dad cared for my mother for a long time while they worked. Dad proved what a remarkable and great man he was down the stretch but finally succumbed to brain cancer.

My brothers and sister-in-law did their best to take care of mom, but it came at a price. Caregiving for a dementia patient is an indescribable horror I would not wish on my worst enemy. You must watch somebody you love wilt away, little by little until dementia wipes away huge chunks of their personality.

Living away, my wife and I visited when possible. We saw how mom deteriorated, but also the effect caregiving had on my father and brothers. It was like watching a train wreck over and over, each time getting worse and helpless to prevent it.

Watching Alzheimer's takedown, my strong-willed mother and others bruised my soul. My writing shifted initially to learn about Alzheimer's, but the more learned, the more I cringed.

The cold hard facts rendered me speechless. Over 5.8 million Americans, and 44 million people worldwide, suffer Alzheimer's. No cure. Just a devastating and expensive slow march towards an agonizing end.

Not content to kill, Alzheimer's tortured Mom for years before killing her. It robbed her memory and damaged her brain, where she repeated herself in a continuous loop, each time thinking she was saying it the first time. As the disease advanced, the neurological disorder destroyed her mind and body.

Seeing dementia take down that tough old bird rattled me. While I could not bring back my mother, I dedicate my life to researching and writing about dementia 8-12 hours per day, six or seven days per week.

I tackled Alzheimer's to learn everything I could about the brute and determine how I and others might prevent it and other noncommunicable diseases. Having written on nutrition and advocated health in Washington, I already had a clue but determined to figure out how to prevent Alzheimer's. But I needed to know more, much more, about this terrorizing neurological disorder.

I learned Alzheimer's was just one of over one-hundred neurological disorders causing dementia. When I searched for a book covering the primary dementias, none existed. Instead, I turned to individual books and again found no books written on several of the most frequent dementias.

In what on the one hand seems like yesterday and the other a lifetime ago, I set out several years ago to write a dementia book covering the 15 most prevalent dementia types. The first to do that, I next wrote books covering each of the 15 most prevalent dementias.

In 2020, I expanded the book covering 15 dementias to 19 dementia types. I also released books on each of the 19 dementias. While proud of these medical firsts, I do not take myself too seriously.

As one of the dozens of scientists, neurologists, researchers, and writers who devote their lives to fighting the war against dementia, I remain humble. I appreciate the individual and combined accomplishments of everybody else in the field.

Nor should any of us get cocky knowing we're losing the war. If we win the war during my lifetime, I will celebrate with hundreds of people worldwide who helped defeat the great beast of our day.

My two-book series break medical ground, and I consider major achievements but remain two among hundreds of significant contributions to the dementia field by people around the globe.

The series provides patients and loved ones a great resource for dementias not covered as extensive as Alzheimer's and the more prevalent types.

By covering the 19 most prevalent dementias, doctors, nurses, and medical professionals benefit from a series covering neurological disorders causing 99% of dementia. The series helps primary care physicians, providers, and nurses who struggle to diagnose dementias with overlapping symptoms.

The series is an organic, evolving work, and each book receives major annual updates. As science uncovers information, we add important data in new editions. We also polish each edition.

We describe the writing goal in three ways:

1. Simplify the language and make it easier for nonscientists to comprehend.
2. Honor the science and facts.
3. Document science and include citations for doctors, nurses, medical researchers, students, and patients.

Our goal is to provide invaluable medical information for professionals, patients, loved ones, and caregivers.

I do not reinvent the wheel but accumulate the best research and teach our readers a better understanding of Alzheimer's and the other 18 primary dementia types.

Among the worst news is one of our loved ones has dementia. A killer disease with no cure frightens the bravest souls.

This medical condition destroys, not just the inflicted, but their loved ones. Besides the patient, nobody suffers more than voluntary caregivers. Watching a mother, father, brother, sister, wife, or husband suffering dementia brutalizes the soul.

I study dementia year around to write and release annual updates to honor people—including my mother—taken by Alzheimer's or one of the other primary dementias.

Modest book royalties are the only compensation, as I accept no money from corporations to promote their product. Nor do I have an ax to grind with anybody in the medical profession.

Having written 100 plus books over four decades, I am thankful to readers for collectively providing me a decent income. However, now in my sixties, I care little about riches and fame.

Who is the reading audience?

The audience falls into five categories.

Those Diagnosed with Dementia

If doctors diagnose you with dementia, my heart goes out to you. You're in for a long battle. Do yourself a favor and focus on slowing the disease and extending the quality of life. One word of caution, the books in this series speak to not only patients, but also families, doctors, students, nurses, and caregivers. Many of those diagnosed with dementia appreciate and benefit from the books, but some find some of the material too disturbing. I intend to write books exclusively for patients but must finish the work related to this series first. While there is not anything too shocking, I wrote the material for a wide audience, meaning I am not always speaking to patients specifically. I promise to personalize an edition for patients and loved ones after finishing this series. By shining a light on all 19 primary dementia types, I hope to help the medical community better distinguish and diagnose neurological disorders.

Loved Ones of Those Diagnosed

If doctors diagnose a loved one with dementia, he or she needs you more than ever. Depending on the type, dementia causes behavioral problems, memory issues, motor decline, and other psychological and physical disorders. The learning curve is steep and changes as one moves from one stage to the next. As with those with dementia, I warn families these books provide a technical overview, and the emphasis is not always on the emotional aspect. If you want to learn about dementias, this series is a great option. If you're looking more for emotional support, there are more appropriate books. I also plan to write a book specifically for families once fulfilling responsibilities for this series.

Medical Professionals

If you are a medical professional interested in studying the dementias, the series covers the dementias responsible for 99% of dementia. While neurologists probably already know the 19 primary dementias, the books provide a quick overview and reference for primary care physicians, nurses, other medical professionals, and students. I also include citations so you can continue your investigation beyond the book's scope.

Volunteer & Professional Caregivers

If you are a dementia caregiver, you are also in for a long, difficult march. Dementia patients demand 24/7 care in later stages, requiring help to go to the bathroom, bathing, and other basic daily functions. While this series is not written solely for caregiving, caregivers benefit by gaining a better understanding of each dementia, their symptoms, and progression.

Anybody Wanting to Learn About A Disease That Strikes 1 Of 6 Americans, And 1 Of 3 Seniors

The series benefits anybody who wants to gain an intermediate understanding of the 19 dementias.

Series' First Lesson

Doctors, like teachers, are part of a sacred profession. **Nothing I say or write replaces your need for a competent doctor!** Nor does any criticism of the profession diminish my respect and admiration for the best.

I detest the worst teachers who fail students and society but love and respect the best. Society would crumble without the most devoted and competent teachers.

Similar, I abhor incompetent, greedy doctors who fail patients and society, but love and respect the best.

The profession must weed out incompetent, uncaring, corrupt doctors, and medical personnel. Every profession has a percentage of bad apples, but within the medical profession, they are cancerous!

Nothing good I write about the medical profession includes incompetent, uncaring doctors, researchers, nurses, etc. And nothing bad I write targets the best.

The series criticizes the profession when deserved, but the first lesson in this series: **Find a competent doctor!** If you have one, count your blessings. If not, find one.

Just as one can learn outside the classroom, we live in a blessed age where medical information is available for anybody on the internet. Such information serves us well, but do not—for a minute-think it replaces the need for a competent, devoted doctor.

The Wrong Doctors

Let me begin this section by saying I love and respect quality doctors, nurses, researchers, and medical professionals from the bottom of my heart and the fullness of my mind.

However, this section is not about what's right in the medical profession.

Glorified idiots, bad doctors are dangerous parasites who dishonor a noble profession. Smart enough to finish medical school, but greedy or flawed beyond redemption, they are like priests working for the devil. Among the worse members of society are doctors motivated by greed or limited by incompetence. Walking parasites!

The Wrong Doctors + Big Pharm + Big Insurance + Big Hospital = Expensive & Inadequate Health Care

Over the past few decades, Big pharmaceuticals, Big Insurance, and their political puppets appointed doctors sanctioned drug dealers. Entrusting the worse doctors with such powers produces little or no better results than assigning the task to a thug on the worst corner in America.

The worst doctors who hand out drugs like candy serve nobody's purpose but their own and **Big Pharm**.

Not an indictment of the entire profession, but unfortunately, **Big Insurance** dictates the typical office visit includes a quick examination and one or more prescriptions. The approach is not based on good science and runs counter to everything science teaches us.

What About Some Tough Love?

The one thing people today do not want is what we often need most, tough love. People want everything sugarcoated and easy.

The problem is most of the time; life is neither sweet nor easy.

What patients need much of the time is not an alleged "magic pill," but instead tough love. Doctors must learn nutrition and teach patients to eat healthier, exercise more, and get 7-8 hours of sleep per night. Like it or not, this is part of modern medicine. Showing up and passing out pills all day is not preventing Alzheimer's and other dementias, nor curing them.

Medical professionals must lead by example and embrace the science of nutrition, exercise, and sleep. If a healthy diet and exercise are the two cornerstones to health, the third is sleep.

The average person needs few or no drugs if they practice healthy habits.

Any doctor who does not vigorously advocate a balanced whole food diet, exercise most days of the week, and 7-8 hours' sleep per night neglects their duty and

Instead, too many doctors ignore the three cornerstones of health and are content to write their patients unnecessary and potentially dangerous prescriptions for the rest of their lives. 100%

emphasis on treating symptoms with drugs, which often require more drugs to counter the side effects, is producing disastrous results. To be the best doctor, one must also emphasize prevention.

Failed Drug Trials

None of the drug trials have produced even one drug that cures Alzheimer's and other dementias. While science has failed to produce any effective dementia drugs, scientific studies prove we can do much by practicing healthy habits to slow or reduce our dementia risk.

The Medical Profession Must Think Outside the Box

The hopeless circle of failed drug trials demands we think outside the box or, as neurologist David Perlmutter advocates, expand the box. He and other neurologists deserve credit for recognizing medicine is failing the dementia war and rocking the boat of conventional wisdom. I must not agree with every point "maverick" neurologists like David Perlmutter, Dale Bredesen, and Deepak Chopra make to respect them for turning conventional wisdom on its head.

Conventional wisdom is losing the Alzheimer's and dementia war!

Not Anti-doctors or Anti-drugs

I am not anti-doctors or anti-drugs and do not understand those who insist neither are needed. I revere competent doctors who practice and advocate the three cornerstones of health. I also recognize the polio vaccine and many other drugs as nothing short of miraculous.

But, my love for what is right about the medical profession will not silence me about what is wrong. And, pretending drugs are the answer to defeating Alzheimer's or dementia is a colossal failure.

You cannot **"do no harm"** and write prescription drugs at the volume of the average doctor.

Choose A Doctor with The Same Care as You Do A Spouse

Find a competent, dedicated, caring, experienced, informed, ethical doctor who listens and respects your opinion, and writes prescriptions as a **LAST RESORT**.

Without the right doctor, you are at the mercy of a profit-oriented health system that seldom puts the patient's interests first, second, or third.

Nothing I say or write in these books or elsewhere means you should not see a doctor, stop taking your medication, or otherwise undermine the medical profession's ability to diagnose and treat any medical symptoms you might experience.

Find a good doctor you trust with your life and ask him or her pointed questions concerning your health and any treatment they recommend.

Outside the Bubble

I challenge the medical profession where necessary, just as I criticize Congress and the United States government for their mistakes or shortcomings. My brief career as a Congressional staffer taught me how difficult it is to maintain one's focus inside the bubble.

Seeing the big picture is no less challenging inside the medical bubble motivated by profit.

Profiteers fund too many studies to promote their product or discredit somebody else's. Blatant self-interests taint studies and confuse the public. Such contradictory studies confuse and make it impossible for the average person to understand which studies to believe.

I respect ethical, competent, dedicated, and hardworking nurses, doctors, and other medical personnel. As much as I criticize what is wrong within the profession, I cannot praise the majority of medical professionals often enough. Getting quality medical care when we need it is one of life's greatest blessings.

Nor do I object to medical-related businesses making a reasonable profit in return for needed medical supplies and services.

Nor should any competent and ethical medical professionals object to anybody challenging medical incompetence and profiteers.

Trust Thy Doctor

The right doctor does not discriminate between physical and mental diseases, so hold back nothing if you or a loved one exhibits symptoms.

If you lack the right doctor, find the right one. Outside you and the daily habits you establish, nobody is more important than your doctor for your health. You must be able to tell him or her medical information you might be reluctant to tell your closest confidant in life.

Remember, doctors too often misdiagnose dementia. Once the symptoms of these deadly dementias set in, you need to see your doctor, provide them with all the information about your problem, and help the specialists reach the correct diagnosis.

Because no tests exist for most dementias, doctors order tests and go through a process of elimination until reaching a diagnosis based on the symptoms you report. The more information you provide, the better the chance of a quick and accurate diagnosis.

Adopt healthy lifestyle choices to prevent dementia when possible, but the next best option is to diagnose it early, to confront it head-on, and take steps to slow the disease. Once dementia hits, it's often possible to postpone the advanced stages. If you've seen a loved one inflicted with dementia, you understand how precious a year, a month, a week, or day is once the storm aims at you or a loved one.

Prolonging life in late-stage dementia without a cure amounts to cruel and unusual punishment, but patients, families, and doctors must do everything possible to extend quality of life while possible.

Make certain you have a doctor who believes in prevention and natural cures, but also remember you need their expertise concerning the best that modern medicine offers.

Be Your Nurse!

If you have a loved one, be each other's nurse. If not, be your nurse.

It's more important than ever for you to monitor your blood pressure and make notes of health issues as they arise. We don't go to the doctor every time we develop a symptom or don't feel well, but it's important to keep a medical journal. Write an outline of the problems you experience between visits.

Too often, we march into the physician's office and don't provide a full or accurate representation of our problem. For instance, if you track your blood pressure, you can furnish a pattern rather than a onetime reading. You can also perhaps attribute pikes in your blood pressure to stress taking place in your life.

You should also track other symptoms. Providing thorough information helps doctors eliminate multiple diseases with similar symptoms. When you document all or most of the symptoms that have led to the visit, you provide a competent doctor a clearer picture to develop a hypothesis. These previous unrelated symptoms might help your physician make more sense of what prompted the appointment.

Otherwise, your physician might order the wrong tests or prescribe the wrong drugs. For issues of the brain, you can't be shy or embarrassed about providing your physician with a full portrayal of your problems and symptoms.

Although still stigmatized in some circles, mental illnesses are just as real, and the sufferers are no more the blame, than physical disorders. While we must do everything in our power to avoid or slow mental or physical maladies, the last thing we need to do is embarrass those who are already suffering.

Two Dementia Series

The laborious task to document the primary dementias began as a fifty-page Alzheimer's overview. Two editions later, the 50-page Alzheimer's book turned into 400 pages.

One of the first lessons taught Alzheimer's is only one of the hundreds of diseases responsible for dementia. With inadequate testing, similar symptoms, and other handicaps, the medical community often misdiagnoses the other dementias for Alzheimer's.

My focus broadened from Alzheimer's to a dozen dementias. The only way to make any sense of Alzheimer's or dementia was to study all the primary dementias.

I worked with several neurologists and researchers over the next couple of years and hit every medical library I could hit in person or available online.

After an extensive review, I wrote the first book covering the 15 most prevalent dementia types, which provided the groundwork for two updated dementia series.

The associated *Dementia Types, Symptoms, Stages, & Risk Factors, series* expands the collection by adding amyotrophic lateral sclerosis (ALS), early-onset Alzheimer's disease, amyotrophic lateral sclerosis, corticobasal syndrome, and progressive supranuclear palsy.

Two Dementia Series

Not counting mixed dementia, there are nineteen primary dementia types, which two groundbreaking series covers.

Dementia Types, Symptoms, Stages, & Risk Factors series

1. _Dementia with Lewy Bodies_
2. _Parkinson's Disease Dementia_
3. Corticobasal Syndrome
4. Typical Alzheimer's Disease
5. _Posterior Cortical Atrophy_
6. _Down Syndrome with Alzheimer's_
7. _Limbic-predominant Age-related TDP-43 Encephalopathy (LATE)_
8. Early-onset Alzheimer's
9. _Behavioral Variant Frontotemporal Dementia_
10. Progressive Supranuclear Palsy
11. _Nonfluent Primary Progressive Aphasia_
12. Logopenic Progressive Aphasia
13. _Cortical Vascular Dementia_
14. _Binswanger Disease_
15. _Normal Pressure Hydrocephalus_
16. _Huntington's Disease_
17. _Korsakoff Syndrome_
18. _Creutzfeldt-Jakob Disease_
19. Amyotrophic Lateral Sclerosis

*Not a dementia type, but a combination, mixed dementia is the 20th category important in dementia discussions.

Any disease leading to symptoms is a dementia type. The series breaks medical ground by covering the dementias responsible for over 99% of cases.

Dementia Overview Series

The second series focuses on all the primary dementia types or breaks them down as groups.

2020 Dementia Overview Series

1. Dementia Types, Symptoms, & Stages
2. Lewy Body/Parkinsonism Dementias
3. Vascular Dementia
4. Frontotemporal Dementia (FTD)
5. Alzheimer's Related Dementias
6. Prevent or Slow Dementia

The Best Science in Everyday Language

The text in both series contains American, Australian, British, and other English. I write in American English, but the research comes from the best studies worldwide. Quotes from the UK, Australia, and other English-speaking countries depend on the local dialect. For integrity, I do not edit quotes.

The books include facts and science as they exist. As much as possible, we replace medical jargon with everyday language.

Having explained the series, let's discuss dementia.

I. DEMENTIA

In this section, we discuss dementia.

Dementia is not a disease but a medical condition. Hundreds of diseases and disorders lead to dementia, but percentage-wise, almost all dementia falls under 19 primary dementia categories.

This series is the first to cover all 19 primary dementia types.

In this chapter, we answer the following questions:

- What is dementia?
- What are the 19 primary dementias?
- How prevalent is dementia?
- Who is most likely to get dementia?
- What are the financial costs to individuals, the U.S., and worldwide?

Once we answer these questions and provide a dementia overview, we turn our attention to the subject matter for the rest of the book.

Let's begin by answering the question: What is dementia?

Chapter 1: WHAT IS DEMENTIA?

For centuries, when one got dementia, people described the person in terms like "gone mad," or "lost their mind," or "crazy," or another derogatory term that missed the mark.

While most dementia types attack cognitive skills and cause behavioral disorders, the person is no less a victim than a cancer patient.

Whereas cancer attacks cells and organs, dementia destroys brain neurons.

The brain is complex. One-hundred billion neurons use over 100 trillion synapses and about 100 neurotransmitters to send all the signals to other parts of the brain, organs, and parts throughout the body, allowing us to think, reason, walk, talk, breathe, and do all that makes us human.

When fed, protected, and healthy, neurons perform magic.

The different dementias attack the brain and destroy the communication network responsible for everything our body does. By attacking different parts of the brain, the dementia types cause different disorders.

Let's see how some of the most prestigious American and global medical organizations define Dementia.

Alzheimer's Association Definition

Let's begin with the Alzheimer's Association:

Dementia is an overall term for diseases and conditions characterized by a decline in memory, language, problem-solving, and other thinking skills that affect a person's ability to perform everyday activities. Memory loss is an

*example. Alzheimer's is the most common
cause of dementia[1].*

Dementia is to Alzheimer's, dementia with Lewy bodies, Parkinson's dementia, vascular and the other dementia types what Asia is to China, India, North Korea, South Korea, and the rest of Asia. Alzheimer's is the most prevalent dementia, but each type devastates, and most are death sentences.

Let's turn to the National Institute on Aging (NIH) and see how they define dementia.

National Institute on Aging (NIH)

The National Institute on Aging (NIH) funds many studies and provides researchers invaluable data. How do they define dementia?

*Dementia is the loss of cognitive
functioning – thinking, remembering, and
reasoning – and behavioral abilities to such an
extent that it interferes with a person's daily
life and activities. These functions include
memory, language skills, visual perception,
problem-solving, self-management, and the
ability to focus and pay attention. Some people
with dementia cannot control their emotions,
and their personalities may change. Dementia
ranges in severity from the mildest stage, when
it is just beginning to affect a person's
functioning, to the most severe stage, when the
person must depend completely on others for
basic activities of living[2].*

One of the most important things a person and their loved ones can do when diagnosed with dementia; enjoy what quality time remains.

Early diagnosis, medication, and lifestyle changes can slow the disease and extend quality life. From the point of diagnosis, make the most of each good day or moment.

Let's see how the international community defines dementia.

Alzheimer's Society UK

The Alzheimer's Society is perhaps the UK's most prestigious Alzheimer's organization. They define dementia:

The word 'dementia' describes a set of symptoms that may include memory loss and difficulties with thinking, problem-solving or language. These changes are often small to start with, but for someone with dementia they have become severe enough to affect daily life. A person with dementia may also experience changes in their mood or behaviour[3].

World Health Organization (WHO)

The World Health Organization (WHO) works with global medical organizations and provides researchers a wealth of information. How does WHO define dementia?

Dementia is a syndrome – usually of a chronic or progressive nature – in which there is deterioration in cognitive function (i.e. the ability to process thought) beyond what might be expected from normal ageing. It affects memory, thinking, orientation, comprehension, calculation, learning capacity, language, and judgement. Consciousness is not affected. The impairment in cognitive function is commonly accompanied, and occasionally preceded, by deterioration in emotional control, social behaviour, or motivation[4].

The four organizations provide similar definitions, each emphasizing different points, but none contradicting the others.

Each organization confirms dementia is a broad neurological disorder. Hundreds of pathologies such as Alzheimer's leads to dementia, but 19 primary types cause about 99% of dementia cases. Dementia attacks the brain and causes memory decline, behavior disorders, motor decline, language deterioration, and most types are incurable.

If doctors diagnose you with dementia, you must get past the shock. Time is moving against you, so make the most of it.

As the Alzheimer's Society points out, the symptoms are minor in the beginning. Get your affairs in order, enjoy loved ones, and take part in as many activities as you desire and are able. To some extent, this is your farewell tour. Take advantage!

The disease will stop you or a loved one later, so do not stop living your life in the early stages.

Let's next examine the 19 primary dementia types.

Chapter 2: WHAT ARE THE 19 PRIMARY DEMENTIAS?

Hundreds of medical conditions lead to dementia, but 19 causes up to 99% of cases.

Each dementia type is devastating, most are fatal, and the first symptoms to death is a challenging, heartbreaking, soul-crushing experience. Dementia robs the personalities and functionality of marvelous people a little at a time until they no longer resemble the person they've always been.

19 Dementia Types

This chapter divides the 19 primary dementias into six categories. The first group includes dementias related to Lewy body or Parkinsonism dementia. The second consists of Alzheimer's-related dementia. In the third, we focus on primary progressive aphasia dementias. The fourth contains vascular dementias. The fifth category encompasses the remaining dementias and is called *other dementias.*

Lewy Body/Parkinsonism Related Dementias

1. *Dementia with Lewy Bodies*
2. *Parkinson's Disease Dementia*
3. Corticobasal Syndrome

Alzheimer's Related Dementias

4. Typical Alzheimer's Disease
5. *Posterior Cortical Atrophy*
6. *Down Syndrome with Alzheimer's*
7. *Limbic-predominant Age-related TDP-43 Encephalopathy (LATE)*
8. Early-onset Alzheimer's

Frontotemporal Lobar Degeneration Related Dementias

9. *Behavioral Variant Frontotemporal Dementia*
10. Progressive Supranuclear Palsy

Primary Progressive Aphasia Related Dementias

11. <u>Nonfluent Primary Progressive Aphasia (nfvPPA)</u>
12. <u>Logopenic Progressive Aphasia (LPA)</u>

Vascular Dementia

13. <u>Cortical Vascular Dementia</u>
14. <u>Binswanger Disease</u>

Other Dementias

15. <u>Normal Pressure Hydrocephalus</u>
16. <u>Huntington's Disease</u>
17. <u>Korsakoff Syndrome</u>
18. <u>Creutzfeldt-Jakob Disease</u>
19. <u>Amyotrophic Lateral Sclerosis</u>

Chapter 3: WHO IS MOST LIKELY TO GET DEMENTIA?

In this chapter, we explore who is most likely to get dementia. Most know people with dementia are old, but some people are born with dementia, others get it as infants, and the disease attacks people in every age group.

There are risk factors that affect everybody. Examples include a poor diet, lack of exercise, diabetes, obesity, high blood pressure, and factors under and beyond our control.

In this chapter, we focus on risk factors affecting specific groups of people who suffer higher rates.

The research pointed to age, race, and sex, where dementia seems to discriminate. Let's review the science for each.

Age

Age is the obvious risk factor. We know because of science and our observations.

So associated with the elderly, many believe dementia only strikes older people. However, dementia strikes all ages and demographics, including newborns and infants.

According to Stanford University Medical School, "The risk of Alzheimer's disease, vascular dementia, and several other dementias goes up significantly with advancing age[5]."

None of us enjoy aging. We must work harder and harder to slow aging, and no matter how well we do, none of us will make it much past 100 years. The better we take care of ourselves, the higher chance we have of living a quality life into our eighties or nineties.

Remember, aging does not destroy our cognitive abilities. Bad habits do! I stress this point because each of us can slow the aging process through healthy habits.

As people age, however, our dementia risks increase.

A Journal of Neurology, Neurosurgery, & Psychiatry study concluded[6]:

> In the age group 65–69 years, there are more than two new cases per 1000 persons every year. This number increases almost exponentially with increasing age, until over the age of 90 years, out of 1000 persons, 70 new cases of dementia can be expected every year.

As we stress in our book on prevention, there is actual age and real age. We determine one's actual age by the day and year born, whereas weight, blood pressure, blood sugar, cholesterol, diet, how often you work out, and several other important factors govern our real age.

Unless genes or an accident prevents us, our real age should be lower than our actual age. Those who practice bad habits, however, raise their real age ten years or more than their actual age.

When our real age is lower than our actual age, we lower our risks for dementia and other diseases. When our real age is higher than our actual age, we increase risks for dementia, heart disease, cancer, and all major diseases.

Let's next review if race plays a role in dementia.

Race

African Americans and blacks in western countries suffer more than their share of racism.

The United States has abused too many citizens since its creation, but none more than Native Americans and African Americans.

But, does dementia also discriminate against them?

According to AARP, African Americans are 64% more likely to get dementia than non-Hispanic whites[7].

Kaiser Permanente Study

Researchers in another study examined data from 274,000 Kaiser Permanente patients over 14 years. They found the highest rate of dementia for African Americans and Native Americans[8].

Dementia Risk Per 1,000 People

27   African Americans

22   Native Americans

20   Latinos and Pacific Islanders

19   White Americans

15   Asian-Americans

Does dementia love Asian and European-Americans and hate African and Native-Americans?

Dementia is as evil as the worst bigot, but dementia is not a bigot.

African Americans experience higher rates of diabetes. African Americans and Native Americans suffer a higher level of stress, poverty, and disenfranchisement. Both cultures also struggle with their people's history in European-America and endure a greater level of bigotry and more obstacles to succeeding in modern America.

On the flip side, Asian Americans and whites have lower obesity and diabetes rates, eat a more balanced diet, faceless bigotry, are more affluent, educated, and successful in modern America.

We need more studies to confirm the exact causes of higher dementia incidence in the African and Native American populations. Higher stress and diabetes in their communities are prime suspects.

Jennifer Manly, Columbia University, Taub Institute for Research on Alzheimer's disease, and Aging Brain spoke to Reuters about the inequities.

> *There are huge disparities in dementia that are confronting this nation, and this will translate into an enormous burden on families if we don't address this. We need to prioritize research that uncovers the reasons for these disparities and more research should include racially and ethnically diverse people[9].*

Are African British at a greater risk for Dementia?

In the United Kingdom, black women are 25% more likely than white women, and black men 28% more likely than white men to get dementia[10].

Reluctance to Take Part in Dementia Studies

African Americans and Native Americans are also less trustful of studies. Too often in the past, a bigoted establishment treated African Americans and Native Americans like lab rats.

The awful past makes the average African American reluctant to take part in studies that might help us figure out how to lower the rates.

Native Americans are also distrustful of the United States government and the "white man's studies," as one group from the Cherokee Reservation in North Carolina told me.

I understand both ethnic groups' skepticism. As somebody with ancestors who died and survived the Trail of Tears, and who married a black woman (30+ years), nobody must convince me of the tainted American history. I have read about the past and viewed enough with my own eyes to know the sins of America's past, either haunt or still torment today.

But, the Studies are Necessary!

I call on African Americans and Native Americans to take part in dementia studies. The studies today have greater safeguards than the past and face much more scrutiny.

Dementia is a death sentence!

Worse than the average killer, never content to kill and move on, dementia is a sadist. Dementia destroys the mind and body, little by little, robbing one's personality, dignity, mind, body, and everything that makes a person unique.

If African Americans and Native Americans refuse to participate in dementia studies, fatal neurological disorders will continue to strike them worse than other ethnic groups.

Please consider two facts.

If you do not have dementia, researchers do not subject you to drug trials but accumulate data to determine which habits increase and decrease one's risks.

If doctors diagnose you with dementia, trials represent your last best chance to win what is otherwise a losing battle.

What Role does Poverty Play?

Although not listed as a dementia risk factor, poverty

increases one's risk for almost every significant disease. Those at the bottom must worry where the next meal is coming, if somebody might mug (or kill) them when leaving the house, and a laundry list of stress the average citizen seems oblivious.

Beller Health calls for more research to determine if Native American, African American, and African British citizens have higher dementia rates as a general population, or if poverty drives these numbers. We need to know whether the number also applies to middle-and upper-class African Americans and Native Americans who eat healthily, exercise, do not abuse alcohol, avoid tobacco, and do not abuse prescription or illicit drugs.

Native American, African American, and African British citizens suffer a higher percentage of poverty than other demographics in the US and UK.

Rather than race, such factors as poverty, bigotry, and lack of opportunities might drive these numbers.

I reached out to several organizations, including the VA, to conduct a large-scale study to determine what role poverty plays in dementia. Most organizations greeted my request with enthusiasm, and I hope one or more soon back the study.

All we know for certain is poverty in the industrial world causes a much greater level of stress and other hardships than the rest of the population. WHO reported that about 60% of dementia cases occur in the poorest half of countries[11].

Age and ethnicity are dementia risk factors. What about sex?

Sex

Dementia strikes older people, African Americans, Native Americans, and African British in greater numbers than the rest of the population. Does one's gender increase or decrease one's odds?

How Many Women have Dementia?

According to the Alzheimer's Association, women represent two-thirds of people living with Alzheimer's, and 13 million women suffer dementia or are caring for somebody who does[12].

Of the 820,000 people living with dementia in the UK, females account for 61 percent[13].

Of the 50 million people living with dementia worldwide[14], women represent 65 percent[15].

Key points:

- Women represent two-thirds of Alzheimer's cases.
- Females account for 65% of dementia cases.

Is dementia just another woman-hating predator?

Does Alzheimer's & Most Dementia Strike Women in Greater Numbers?

While the two key numbers suggest dementia is a rampaging woman-abusing murderer, the answer is not so simple.

While women represent two-thirds of Alzheimer's cases and 65% of dementia cases, there are 19 primary dementia types.

Some dementias attack men in greater numbers and much harder than females. The dementias we know attack men in greater ratios include[16]:

- Parkinson's dementia (Lewy body dementia)
- Dementia with Lewy bodies (Lewy body dementia)
- Post-Stroke dementia (Vascular dementia)
- Multi-infarct dementia (Vascular dementia)
- Binswanger Disease(Vascular dementia)
- Normal pressure hydrocephalus
- Behavioral variant frontotemporal dementia
- Primary Progressive Aphasia (Frontotemporal dementia)
- Chronic traumatic encephalopathy
- HIV-related cognitive impairment
- Amyotrophic lateral sclerosis

From the data about the 19 primary dementias, at least eleven attack men in greater numbers. Data is not available for Creutzfeldt-Jakob disease, Wernicke-Korsakoff Syndrome, LATE, and Down syndrome with Alzheimer's disease. The remaining dementias strike both genders in similar numbers. When the authorities release more information, we will update this section.

If a minimum of 11 of 19 dementia types strike men in greater numbers than women, how can 68% of people living with dementia be women?

Alzheimer's accounts for 60-80% of dementia, and two-thirds of people with Alzheimer's are women.

When we say dementia attacks, women, 65% to 35% men, we distort the picture. I call on the medical community to provide greater clarity. More precise, we should warn women to represent two-thirds of total Alzheimer's cases, but stress a minimum of 11 of 19 dementia types strike men in greater numbers.

Treating dementia and Alzheimer's as interchangeable terms is misleading. There are 19 primary dementias and 11 or more attack men in greater numbers. If we exclude Alzheimer's and focus on the other 18 primary dementia types, they attack men by far greater percentages.

With that stipulation, let's explore why Alzheimer's and some dementias attack women more than men.

Why Does Alzheimer's & Dementia Strike Women in Greater Numbers Than Men?

In part, unique burdens & responsibilities explain the disparity.

Women still fight today for equality. Like Native Americans, African Americans, and African British, the average woman carries burdens; the average man is clueless.

To be a woman, one fights for equality from birth in a "man's world," as the song and tradition attest. Among things unique to women:

- Menstrual cycles (ranging from mild to horrendous)
- Childbirth
- Menopause

Being a guy is also difficult, but there's no denying women are born with unique responsibilities and burdens.

As an aunt once retorted, if they live long enough, every woman suffers menstrual cycles until menopause "tortures it out."

Women Live Longer

Women outlive men in the United States and worldwide.

Worldwide, the average man lives to age 69.8, while the average woman lives 74.2 years[17]. These are the average numbers, so they fluctuate from region to region and country to country.

Let's see how these numbers compare to the United States.

American Comparisons

The CDC reports the average American male lives 76 years, compared to the average American woman who lives 81 years[18].

Why Do Women Live Longer Than Men?

Although women live longer, this might result because more men abuse alcohol, tobacco, and drugs, get less sleep, work in more hazardous jobs, suffer greater casualties in war, and take unnecessary risks.

The lead author of a study published in the *British Medical Journal*, Australian neuropsychiatrist Richard Cibulskis, confirmed some of my suspicions.

> *Men are much more likely to die from preventable and treatable non-communicable diseases, such as {ischemic} heart disease and lung cancer, and road traffic accidents[19].*

Global population expert, Dr. Perminder Sachdev, confirmed my other suspicions in an interview with *Time*.

"Men are more likely to smoke, drink excessively and be overweight," Sachdev said. "They are also less likely to seek medical help early, and, if diagnosed with a disease, they are more likely to be non-adherent to treatment." Sachdev also pointed out, "men are more likely to take life-threatening risks and to die in car accidents, brawls or gunfights[20]."

Although nature perhaps installed a natural order to preserve the female population, men's reckless nature might account for the five years difference in life expectancy between the genders.

It will interest to see if the numbers change as more women become more like men. Women are assuming greater roles in war, law enforcement, and other areas where even men with healthy habits have fallen. As the societal lines between men and women blur, the difference in life expectancy should fall.

In all honorable fields of life, women should go for it. Never has there been a better time to prove the equality of the sexes.

As far as men's bad habits, my hope is women continue to show better judgment and exercise greater restraint. Women will never prove their equality by emulating men's worse habits or trying to outdo us in the stupid department.

The best men and women rise on similar foundations. However, the worst men and women also share a foundation. My hope for humans getting our act together soon hinges on the average woman being better than the average man.

Love yourselves for your unique feminine qualities. Be equal, but please do not confuse out-drinking, out-smoking, out-drugging, acting more reckless, and stupid than men with being equal. We need fewer men like that, not more women!

Chapter 4: DEMENTIA COSTS & PREVALENCE

In this chapter, we review dementia prevalence and costs to governments, the world, caregivers, and patients.

How Many People Worldwide Suffer Dementia?

According to the World Health Organization (WHO), over 50 million people suffer dementia worldwide, with 10 million new cases each year[21].

How Many Americans Have Dementia?

In the United States, 5.8 million Americans live with dementia[22], with Alzheimer's representing 70% of cases.

Let's check the UK dementia numbers.

How Many People in The UK Have Dementia?

According to the Alzheimer's Society, 850,000 people in the UK live with dementia[23].

Alzheimer's Society reports that about 70% of those living in UK care homes suffer dementia.

The numbers show Americans, British, and global citizens suffering high rates of dementia. Let's see which countries' dementia strikes the hardest.

Which Countries Have the Highest Dementia Rate?

Per World Atlas, the following ten countries suffer the highest dementia rate of deaths per 100,000 people[24]:

1. Finland
2. USA
3. Canada
4. Iceland
5. Sweden
6. Switzerland
7. Norway
8. Denmark
9. The Netherlands
10. Belgium

As we review the list, per population, dementia strikes Americans in greater numbers than any country but Finland.

Why?

There are several explanations:

- Over two-thirds of Americans are obese or overweight.
- The other countries on the list also suffer higher obesity levels than most countries not on the list.
- Because of weight issues, the countries in question suffer high rates of diabetes and high blood pressure, both dementia risk factors.
- Americans consume more prescription drugs than people worldwide. While there is no data to confirm, I suspect the other countries on the list

also have greater access and use more prescription drugs than poorer countries.

- They load the western diet with salt, sugar, and white processed flours.
- The average person in western countries lives longer than those in poorer nations.
- We will add other factors once data becomes available.
- People live longer in these countries than most not on the list (the older one lives, the greater the dementia risk)

Another explanation is more misdiagnosis and no-diagnosis in poorer countries around the world. Obesity and other risk factors are also less of a problem in developing countries.

I recommend global researchers compare the ten countries on this list. By viewing the similarities between the ten, we might better pinpoint the cause for Alzheimer's and the other dementias.

If we can figure out what the citizens from the ten nations are doing wrong, we can find the cause and means of preventing dementia. While I pointed to some of the most obvious risk factors, the most important common risk factor from the ten nations might be something unexpected.

Let's now examine dementia costs.

Dementia Costs

In this chapter, we analyze dementia costs. We examine the United States and global costs, then provide estimated costs per family.

What Does Dementia Cost the United States?

More than the entire economies of Finland and 166 other countries, dementia costs the United States $277 billion per year.

What Does Dementia Cost Worldwide?

Getting credible global numbers proves difficult, if not impossible, in any medical research. Often, the best source is the World Health Organization (WHO). They collect data from around the world and are an essential source for medical researchers.

Getting accurate dementia numbers in richer countries is difficult. In the United States and the UK, black people hesitate to take part in dementia studies or to seek medical attention for symptoms.

In richer countries, there are still too many misdiagnoses.

Thus, if we cannot get ironclad numbers in the United States, the United Kingdom, and the industrial nations, the task proves even more difficult for developing countries.

If the United States and the United Kingdom have difficulty convincing black citizens to seek medical attention for dementia symptoms, the third world faces even greater obstacles.

In the third world, most areas do well to offer their citizens basic medical care. With no urine or blood test, many regions lack resources for CAT scans, MRIs, and other expensive imaging equipment to make a diagnosis.

Without urine or blood tests, diagnosing dementia costs more than low-income people with inadequate or no insurance can afford in the richest countries.

In the United States and industrial nations, doctors often misdiagnose the other 19 primary dementias for Alzheimer's or each other.

Expecting doctors in many third world nations to diagnose dementia with inferior or no equipment is to expect miracles. If it overwhelms medical professionals in the wealthier nations, we often expect third world doctors to perform miracles. What amazes is they often do!

However, no matter how well the average third world doctor treats typical medical conditions, even if trained, impoverished circumstances deny them the necessary equipment to diagnose dementia early, if at all. My comments are not criticism.

The average doctor's job is not to diagnose or treat dementia, but they must recognize symptoms and refer the patient to neurologists. Primary care physicians are the first line of defense.

North, south, east, west, dementia overwhelms.

Having discussed the limitations, let's examine the data. While the numbers are ballpark figures, landing in the park is the keystone to estimation. In most cases, the real numbers are much higher.

According to the *World Alzheimer's Report,* global dementia costs a minimum of $1 trillion per year, and experts predict it will reach $2 trillion by 2030 if we find no cure[25].

Authorities should release new numbers over the next year, and we will update this section. The *Alzheimer's Report* global cost estimations do not include informal care costs.

The Alzheimer's Report concluded:

> *Direct medical care costs account for*
> *roughly 20% of global dementia costs, while*
> *direct social sector costs and informal care*

costs each account for roughly 40%. The relative contribution of informal care is greatest in the African regions and lowest in North America, Western Europe and some South American regions, while the reverse is true for social sector costs.

Whatever the real up-to-date costs, we must take action to reduce the burden on individuals and nations. If we do not invest in independent research to develop an effective urine or blood test, cure, and vaccine for each dementia type, the costs will smother economies throughout the world. The costs will cripple developing countries and destabilize the wealthiest.

We have no choice but to invest more in dementia research. No matter which country you live, your economy, security, and the health of your nation rides on us finding a cure or vaccine.

As a scientist, I find it disturbing climate change and independent dementia research are not major priorities. Most governments, businesses, and individuals who can afford to fund dementia remain MIA in the war against dementia.

Before we conclude this section, let's examine the dementia statistics side-by-side in the table below.

DEMENTIA STATISTICS

This table focuses on the number of people with dementia and the number of deaths per 100,000 among the nations chosen for comparison.

NATION	# OF PEOPLE WITH DEMENTIA	DEMENTIA DEATHS PER 100,000 PEOPLE	TOTAL COSTS (US DOLLARS)
Australia	447,115	29.61	$15 billion
Brazil	1 million +	10.71	$16.45 billion
Canadian	747,000	37.30	$10.4 billion
China	16.93 million	19.87	$69 billion
France	1.2 million	30.84	$37.91 billion
Germany	1.5 million	16.99	$57.57 billion
India	4 million	14.57	$28.38 billion
Italy	1.4 million	19.81	$29.96 billion
Japan	4.6 million	7.22	$14.8 billion
Mexico	800,000	3.62	Not available
Spain	800.000+	29.23	$19.98 million
Netherlands	280,000	39.37	$4.44 million
United States	5.8 million	44.41	$290 billion
United Kingdom	850,000	49.18	$26.3 billion

Sources: World Health Rankings[26], Alzheimer's Europe[27], NATSIM[28], Alzheimer's Society[29], Brain Test[30]

Other sources cited in the chapter.

The table comes from my book <u>2020 Dementia Overview</u>, which covers cost and prevalence among comparative nations in greater detail.

Let's next discuss the dementia costs for caregivers.

What Does Dementia Cost Volunteer Caregivers?

Although 41% make less than $50,000, American voluntary caregivers devote a minimum of 18.4 billion hours per year to dementia patients.

Worth $232 billion per year, we underrate the voluntary caregiving heroes in our fight against dementia. This total does not include lost wages for the voluntary caregiver.

According to the Northwestern Mutual C.A.R.E. Study, 67% of voluntary caregivers must cut their living to help pay for the patient's medical care, and 57% end up experiencing financial problems[31].

Adding to the costs of voluntary caregivers, they often end up sick themselves. Caring for loved ones with dementia bankrupts many.

In the early stages, the loved one can still perform most of their daily tasks but will require 24/7 care once the symptoms advance.

Imagine putting your life on hold for years to care, bathe, feed, protect, and take such a heavy load on your shoulders.

Millions of dementia families face the dilemma where the husband and wife both must work in most families to get by. You work as a couple to build stability in your own family, and then, boom, doctors diagnose one of you with dementia.

What Does Dementia Cost Dementia Patients?

When we say patient, past a certain stage in the disease, we refer to family or loved ones. A person who cannot perform daily tasks cannot manage finances, even if they have any left.

Too often, the costs drive entire families into bankruptcy because of dementia costs for a member.

Authorities estimate the average cost per dementia patient is $341,840, with families expected to cover 70 percent.

The costs devastate the average family in the industrial nations.

How are they supposed to afford it in developing countries where the average citizen makes less than one-thousand American dollars per year?

Dementia Recap

Although your dementia research has just begun, you now have a decent overview of Dementia.

In Chapter One, we explored dementia. We turned to several top dementia or medical organizations and compared their definitions.

Chapter two explained Alzheimer's is to dementia what China is to Asia. We listed the 19 dementias. They include:

1. *Dementia with Lewy Bodies*
2. *Parkinson's Disease Dementia*
3. Corticobasal Syndrome
4. Typical Alzheimer's Disease
5. *Posterior Cortical Atrophy*
6. *Down Syndrome with Alzheimer's*
7. *Limbic-predominant Age-related TDP-43 Encephalopathy (LATE)*
8. Early-onset Alzheimer's
9. *Behavioral Variant Frontotemporal Dementia*
10. Progressive Supranuclear Palsy
11. *Nonfluent Primary Progressive Aphasia*
12. Logopenic Progressive Aphasia
13. *Cortical Vascular Dementia*
14. *Binswanger Disease*
15. *Normal Pressure Hydrocephalus*
16. *Huntington's Disease*
17. *Korsakoff Syndrome*
18. *Creutzfeldt-Jakob Disease*
19. Amyotrophic Lateral Sclerosis

Although most the dementia types share similar symptoms, enough to cause misdiagnosis, each has its unique pathology and symptoms.

In chapter three, we explored dementia prevalence in the United States, the UK, and worldwide.

Chapter four examined who is most likely to get dementia. We found Native Americans (those who greeted the first Europeans), and black citizens in the United States and the UK are more likely to get dementia than their white or Asian counterparts.

We also explored the women to men ratio. Women represent two-thirds of Alzheimer's and over sixty percent of dementia cases. We pointed out the Alzheimer's figure skews the dementia numbers because men are more likely to get a minimum of 11 of the 19 primary dementia types.

Chapter four explored the US, UK, global, patient, family, and voluntary caregivers' dementia costs. The staggering numbers are almost as frightening as the medical disorder itself.

We borrowed the following table from *2020 Dementia Overview.*

Dementia Costs & Prevalence

NATION	# OF PEOPLE WITH DEMENTIA	DEMENTIA DEATHS PER 100,000 PEOPLE	TOTAL COSTS (US DOLLARS)
Australia	447,115	29.61	$15 billion
Brazil	1 million +	10.71	$16.45 billion
Canadian	747,000	37.30	$10.4 billion
China	16.93 million	19.87	$69 billion
France	1.2 million	30.84	$37.91 billion
Germany	1.5 million	16.99	$57.57 billion
India	4 million	14.57	$28.38 billion
Italy	1.4 million	19.81	$29.96 billion
Japan	4.6 million	7.22	$14.8 billion
Mexico	800,000	3.62	Not available
Spain	800.000+	29.23	$19.98 million
Netherlands	280,000	39.37	$4.44 million
United States	5.8 million	44.41	$290 billion
United Kingdom	850,000	49.18	$26.3 billion

Sources: World Health Rankings[32], Alzheimer's Europe[33], NATSIM[34], Alzheimer's Society[35], Brain Test[36]

The table comes from 2020 Dementia Overview, which covers cost and prevalence among comparative nations in greater detail.

After reviewing the conservative numbers, and factoring in an aging population, we concluded we must find a cure before it bankrupts millions of families and overwhelms nations.

II. HUNTINGTON'S DISEASE

Let's turn our attention to Huntington's disease.

Chapter 5: WHAT IS HUNTINGTON'S DISEASE (HD)?

The most prevalent, neurodegenerative malady, Huntington's disease (HD), also called Chronic Progressive Chorea, Degenerative Chorea, HD, Hereditary Chorea, Hereditary Chronic Progressive Chorea, Huntington's Chorea, VEOHD, Very Early Onset Huntington's Disease, and Woody Guthrie's disease, is a fatal genetic disorder that kills brain cells.

Like myotonic muscular dystrophy, Huntington's is an autosomal dominant inheritance disorder and poses the same threat to females and males[37].

If one has a genetic link to dementia, which included everybody with Huntington's disease, it is a death sentence. A genetic link to any devastating disease is frightening.

I must stress not everybody who has a parent with Huntington's will get the disease. "Each child of an affected parent has a 50/50 chance of getting the mutant gene," according to John Hopkins Medical, "and therefore has a 50% chance of inheriting the disease."

Not inheriting the disease also breaks the Huntington's disease cycle, for a child who did not inherit the genetic mutation cannot pass it along to their children.

The U.S. Library of Medicine describes Huntington disease[38] as a "progressive brain disorder that causes uncontrolled movements, emotional problems, and loss of thinking ability (cognition)."

For those familiar, this might sound like Parkinson's disease, but there are clear differences.

Whereas Parkinson's disease is an akinetic-rigid syndrome, Huntington's disease is a trinucleotide repeat disorder. To help

49

distinguish between the diseases, we will define both.

Let's discuss akinetic-rigid syndrome to help distinguish Parkinson's from Huntington's disease.

Akinetic-rigid Syndrome

According to Oxford Medicine, akinetic-rigid syndrome produces, "paucity and slowness of movement accompanied by muscle stiffness and resistance to passive movement. The akinetic–rigid syndrome is typical of idiopathic Parkinson's disease, often described as the syndrome of parkinsonism[39]."

Our focus is Huntington's disease, so let's shift the discussion to trinucleotide repeat disorders.

Trinucleotide Repeat Disorders

A trinucleotide repeat disorder repeats genes, toxifies cells, creates an imbalance, and lays the groundwork.

"When the cause of a disease can be traced to having too many copies of a certain nucleotide triplet in the DNA, the disease is said to be a trinucleotide repeat disorder. Today, there are 14 documented trinucleotide repeat disorders that affect human beings[40]."

Huntington's disease is one of the 14 documented trinucleotide repeat disorders. Huntington's disease repeats the codon CAG, which codes for glutamine, an amino acid.

Now we know what causes Huntington's disease, what akinetic rigid syndrome and trinucleotide repeat disorders are, so let's investigate what age the symptoms manifest.

What Age Does Huntington's Disease Strike?

Unlike most dementias, Huntington's disease strikes people in their prime. Ages 30-50 is when most people find their footing, come into their own, refine their goals, and chase new dreams.

According to the Pathology Department at the University of Pittsburgh Medical Center, on average, Huntington's strikes manifests when somebody is age 40, but strikes people as young as 4 and as old as 84, and the average lifespan from there is 13 years[41].

Within the margin of error, The Alzheimer's Association supports the numbers. Huntington's disease "usually develop between ages 30 and 50," Alzheimer's Association[42] said, "but they can appear as early as age 2 or as late as 80."

Huntington's disease is one of the crueler dementias in two ways:

1. Unlike most dementias, genetics causes Huntington's disease.
2. The primary victims are not towards the end but in the prime of life.

As cruel as the typical Huntington's disease version, there is another even more terrifying.

Juvenile Huntington's (JHD) Disease

Juvenile Huntington's disease (JHD) is the term when symptoms show under age twenty. Less common, juvenile Huntington's disease accounts for 5-10% of Huntington's disease (HD) cases[43].

Once Juvenile Huntington's symptoms manifest, the lifespan

is under ten years, less than half the adult version[44].

Juvenile Huntington's disease symptoms include: "changes in personality, coordination, behavior, speech or ability to learn," according to the Huntington's Disease Society of America. "Physical changes include rigidity, leg stiffness, clumsiness, slowness of movement, tremors, or myoclonus."

Any disease robbing kids' childhood churns my stomach and reminds me how random life is. When dementias strike older people, we grieve and struggle while watching the disease destroy the person we once knew, torture, and kill them.

I cannot say losing a child is harder than losing somebody you've known for six to eight decades; an expression repeated a thousand times every time Juvenile Huntington's takes an infant or teenager. In some ways, it is more difficult to lose somebody you have known, loved, and depended on for decades, your entire life. Losing a loved one, young or old, hurts like hell.

But, when fatal diseases attack children, there is a greater unfairness and leaves behind a lasting sting, creating a void too great to fill. We must prevent or cure this disease!

How Many People have Huntington's Disease?

Please understand any numbers we provide are low because medical authorities often misdiagnose Huntington's disease for Parkinson's or Alzheimer's disease.

How Many Americans have Huntington's disease?

Each year, doctors diagnose 30,000 Americans with Huntington's disease, while over 200,000 are high risk[45].

How do the Americans numbers compare worldwide?

Let's review data by Stanford University to compare how many per million are getting Huntington's disease worldwide per million.

Black South African (.06), Japan (1-4), Hong Kong (3.7), and Finland (6.0) had the lowest incidents per million people.

Let's compare this to Europe (40-100), Northern Ireland (64), South Wales (76.1), Scotland (99.4), and the United States (100) incidents per million people[46].

These are dramatic differences that require more studies to figure out why European populations are much more likely to get Parkinson's disease than Asians or black Africans.

Is it the Western diet, lack of exercise, overuse of chemicals, and other environmental factors? The lack of sun exposure (and Vitamin D deficiencies) from European ancestors who drifted north? Is it because they misdiagnose Huntington's disease more in the third world?

The probable answer is all three, but it requires more studies to confirm. The disproportionate percentage of pale people living in western civilization getting Huntington's suggests a mysterious cause related to divergent evolution from eastern and darker cousins.

While I understand eastern civilization's reluctance to fund Huntington's disease research, I can only scratch my head, trying to rationalize why the western world does not invest greater into independent medical research to find a cure and means to prevent Huntington's disease.

What does Huntington's disease cost?

We divide costs into two categories, national and individual.

Annual Individual Huntington's disease costs

STAGE	ANNUAL COMMERCIAL COSTS	ANNUAL MEDICAID COSTS
Stage 1	$4,947	$3,257
Stage 2	$6,040	$5,670
Stage 3	$22,582	$27,111

Source: PubMed Study[47]

Please note, the numbers are in 2013 dollars and are higher today.

When authorities provide newer data, I will update the numbers in the table.

Once again, we call on hospitals and medical authorities to form a digital link providing continuous updated medical information. We should have instant and accurate data, not aged and estimated numbers.

III. HUNTINGTON'S DISEASE SYMPTOMS & STAGES

Chapter 6: HUNTINGTON'S DISEASE SYMPTOMS

Huntington's disease, like other dementias, is a bully disease. Over the years, the torturous bully strips a person's ability to think, focus, reason, remember, balance, sit, or stand still, and everything that makes them a unique, vibrant individual.

"The hallmark symptom of Huntington's disease," explained Alzheimer's Association, "is uncontrolled movement of the arms, legs, head, face and upper body."

Let's put together a Huntington's symptoms list.

Huntington's disease symptoms list

- anger[48]
- anxiety[49]
- balance and posture trouble[50]
- concentration decline[51]
- convulsions of the head, face, arms, legs, and upper body[52]
- depression[53]
- deteriorating reasoning skills[54]
- impaired thinking[55]
- involuntary jerking[56]
- inability to plan and organize[57]
- irritable[58]
- memory problems[59]
- mood swings[60]
- personality changes
- speaking disturbances[61]
- swallowing disorder[62]
- unsteady gait
- weight loss[63]

Perhaps you noticed the similarities between this list and several other dementias, including Alzheimer's and Parkinson's disease. The similarities create confusion and often cause misdiagnosis.

A doctor must weigh the totality of symptoms, medical history, family history, and order the tests to diagnose Huntington's disease.

Chapter 7: HUNTINGTON'S DISEASE (HD)-RELATED SUICIDE

Let's discuss the elephant in the room. A disturbing topic, but too important to ignore, suicide rates jump far higher in Huntington's disease patients than the general population.

Most of Huntington's patients live their entire lives fearing HD, hoping the symptoms never appear, the diagnosis never comes.

The day arrives. In the period leading up to the diagnosis and at different intervals in the progression, it is vital to address depression and emotional issues.

According to Huntington's Disease Society of America, the suicide rate for people with Huntington's disease is ten times the general population. A more recent study released in *Neurology* found Huntington's patients are twelve times more likely to commit suicide than those without HD.

HD suicide rate climbs up to twenty percent pre-symptomatic patients and during certain stage intervals[64]

The Huntington's Disease Society of America recommends:

> *Monitor depression in the person with HD and ask about suicide regularly, as thoughts about death and suicide can be a part of depression. Suicide is of great concern in HD due to cognitive changes in the brain, including disinhibition and impulsivity[65].*

Patients, families, and medical professionals must understand the hopelessness, despair, and anxiety associated with Huntington's.

Emotional Support

Emotional support goes beyond the book's scope, but

Open up to Confidantes

When a neurological disorder strikes, we need to open up to our inner circle. HD is too difficult a road to travel without people to open up and

Mental Health Professionals

One a neurologist diagnoses you or a loved one with Huntington's disease (HD), find a mental health professional who can help navigate the emotional rollercoaster. Ask the neurologist or call the local Huntington's disease organizations and find one who specializes in HD.

Remove Weapons

Remove all weapons from the house, including any unnecessary medicine. Do not make it easy to follow through o any suicidal thoughts associated with HD induced depression and emotional problems.

If you love life, play it safe. The last any of us need when feeling suicidal is an easy and immediate path. Remove anything from the house making suicide potentially easy or fast.

Dances with Elephants

If doctors diagnose you with Huntington's disease, I recommend you read *Dancing with Elephants*[66] for emotional support and a roadmap on how to live with HD.

When diagnosed with Huntington's disease, Jarem Sawatsky refused to stop living. He turned to his family and developed a spiritual circle to develop a new reality of possibilities. Instead of allowing the idea of HD to defeat him before the severity of symptoms, he became an inspiration for the world.

One must not have HD to benefit from Sawatsky's beautifully-written book, but Huntington's patients in-particular should read how Sawatsky thrived through kindness, laughter, and an inspiring determination to face each day, person, event, challenge, setback, and moment with a positive determination.

This book galvanizes the soul and instills hope and courage. Whether you have HD or not, you should read *Dancing with Elephants.*

These ideas are but few to help fight HD-related emotional issues. Ask your mental health specialist for more ideas. Develop a plan protecting your life during darker moments.

Chapter 8: HUNTINGTON'S STAGES

According to the Stanford University Department of Cardiology, there are five stages to Huntington's disease.

1. Preclinical
2. Early-stage
3. Middle-stage
4. Late-stage
5. Death

Huntington's disease is a journey from preclinical when the mutant gene is present but not yet producing symptoms, to a person's last breath.

Depending on various factors, one lives 10-25 years from the initial symptoms.

Preclinical Huntington's disease

The gene mutation is present, but no obvious symptoms show until reaching early-stage Huntington's.

Some studies suggest somebody during the preclinical stage scores lower on some cognitive tests in the 10-15 years before early-stage development.

A National Institutes of Health-funded study found 9-15 years before early-stage Huntington's; a person performs worse on emotional tests than those who will not get the disease[67].

Preclinical Face-like Object Recognition Impairment

The European Huntington's Disease Network, the Biomedical Research Institute, and other partners released a study in *Cortex* showing

> *In conclusion, premanifest HD participants have a specific visuoperceptual deficit that selectively disrupts the perception of face-like objects as early as 15 years before estimated time to diagnosis. This deficit can be measured as an increased number of errors {in recognition of} face-like object stimulus and as an abolition of the N170 component elicited by face-like objects. The occurrence of selective impairment in face-like object processing in the clinical group emphasizes the need to develop specific instruments to capture early changes in premanifest HD[68].*

We need other studies to confirm the results, but I concur with the study's lead author Saul Martínez-Horta's. We need to expedite the development of specific instruments to gauge specific visuoperceptual deficits in the decade or two before other symptoms manifest.

While drug studies and much of Huntington's disease research focuses on what to do once the symptom officially manifests, we're learning the real war is decades early, even preceding birth.

Instead of placing most of our effort on combatting the disease once it manifests to the point where neurologists can diagnose, we must fight this war on the front lines.

We will return to this topic in the causes and risk factors section. Next, we examine early-stage Huntington's disease.

Huntington's Disease (HD) Stage One

Once diagnosed, it is time to plan for declining cognitive and motor skills. Somebody with later stage Huntington's requires help with daily chores and planning tasks such as finances. For now, one maintains control of most matters.

By early-stage Huntington's, a person develops several symptoms, including involuntary movements.

HD Reach describes Huntington's disease:

> *A diagnosis of HD is made when motor symptoms occur. This is a great time to prepare for a future with HD if not addressed earlier. At this point, the person has normal or mildly reduced workability and might need some help with finances. The HD patient can still live independently and typically experiences minimal impairment in activities and chores. Psychiatric symptoms are intermittent and manageable and emerging motor symptoms might become more identifiable[69].*

Early-stage Huntington's disease is not an easy period, but the quiet before the storm. Trouble is brewing, and symptoms develop. Although not severe enough to make one dependent, the symptoms, especially motor skill decline, becomes a more significant problem as HD develops.

In the beginning, one suffers mild coordination deterioration. More vexing might be involuntary jerking or twitching in the face, fingers, or toes.

HD Stage One Duration

The described motor symptoms transpire over the first year.

Huntington's Disease (HD) Stage Two

Following the motor issues in stage one, stage two brings a set of emotional and cognitive issues.

In stage two, HD often causes significant depression issues. A person becomes irritable and unmotivated, moody, and uninhibited.

Executive skills decline causes struggles to perform complicated tasks. Depending on one's position, executive skills decline might complicate matters. Emotional issues also make remaining in a management role impossible for much longer.

Emotional issues make maintaining relationships laborious and difficult. Too often, people who have emotional disorders retreat an isolate themselves at the time they need people most.

Because of the loss of inhibition, some HD patients experience hypersexuality during this period.

Let's review stage two symptoms.

HD Stage Two Symptoms

- Depression
- Unmotivated
- Irritability
- Loss of inhibition
- Moody
- Trouble maintaining relationships
- Trouble performing complicated tasks
- Hypersexuality (not everybody)

HD Stage Two Duration

The symptoms manifest within two to five years.

Middle-stage Huntington's disease

According to the *Physician's Guide to the Management of Huntington's Disease*, by middle-stage Huntington's:

> *Individuals lose the ability to work or drive and may no longer be able to manage their own finances or perform their own household chores, but will be able to eat, dress, and attend to personal hygiene with assistance. Chorea may be prominent, and people with HD have increasing difficulty with voluntary motor tasks. There may be problems with swallowing, balance, falls, and weight loss. Problem-solving becomes more difficult because individuals cannot sequence, organize, or prioritize information[70].*

The disease is advancing, and our loved one loses their remaining independence.

Huntington's Disease Stage Three

Stage one and two symptoms worsen. Stage three of Huntington's causes clumsiness. Earlier motivation problems become more pronounced.

Stage three HD often causes sexual problems. The most troubling addition in stage three might be a profound paranoia or suspiciousness.

The independence in stages one and two becomes dubious. However, by now, one is to sick to perform significant executive skills, making major financial and other important decisions unadvisable.

If the HD patient has not already turned over significant decisions to a trustworthy person, now is the time to do so. By the end of stage three, the decline comes from several sources, each progressive and devastating.

Huntington's Disease Middle Stage Symptoms

Probable middle stage symptoms include:
- Apathetic
- Anxious
- Balance problems
- Chorea (dancing movements) worsen
- Communication issues
- Decreased sexual appetite
- Falls
- Loss of social skills
- Motor skills decline
- Slow movement

- Swallowing trouble
- Problem-solving decline
- Unclear thinking
- Walking difficulty
- Weight loss

These problems grow progressively worse until we reach the even more challenging stage four.

HD Stage Three Duration

Symptoms occur within six to ten years.

Huntington's Disease Stage Four

By stage four, HD patients suffer tremendous cognitive, motor, emotional, and behavioral decline.

Gripping anything is difficult and frustrating. Life grows more difficult. Walking deteriorates further, making one ever more dependent on others for daily tasks.

Memory loss grows severe. What began as minor now grows more problematic. Similar, stage four reduces executive skills and overall intellect to a fraction of their former capability.

Sleeping grows difficult during stage four, not helping the escalating hallucinations and delusions.

HD Stage Four Duration

Stage four symptoms take ten or more years to materialize.

Huntington's Disease Stage Five

Stage five includes everything covered in stages one through five, only worse.

The end nears.

Late-stage Huntington's defeats a person. Whatever fight they had in the middle-stage now or soon disappears. Apathy replaces depression. Most can still understand, but several severe symptoms overwhelm them.

Between eight and eleven percent of Huntington's patients suffer psychosis, which causes auditory and visual hallucinations.

A person loses control of their organs by late-stage Huntington's, including the bladder and bowel control. By late-stage, the chorea issues from early stages stop or lessons, but symptoms overall turn critical.

Other Late-stage Huntington's Disease symptoms may include:

- Bradykinesia
- Crippling cognitive decline
- Dystonia
- Rigidity
- Severe apathy
- Sleep problems
- Volunteer movement difficulties

HD Stage Five Duration

HD stage five lasts about one year or less.

Additional Stages Sources: Stanford Medical School[71], Columbia University Department of Neurology[72], Huntington's Outreach Project for Education, at Stanford[73],

IV. HUNTINGTON'S DISEASE (HD) RISK FACTORS

When we speak of dementia risk factors, most types pertain to lifestyle choices.

What one eats, how much one exercise, and getting 7.5-8.5 hours sleep per night, not smoking or abusing alcohol, and otherwise practicing healthy habits remains important for those with a genetic HD risk.

However, unlike the majority of dementia, genetics causes Huntington's.

Chapter 9: HUNTINGTON'S DISEASE CAUSE & RISK FACTORS

In this section, we will explore what causes Huntington disease.

Genetics plays a small role in most dementia-related diseases, and the causes remain unknown, but Huntington's disease is an exception.

Genetics is 100% responsible for Huntington disease.

An inherited gene defect causes Huntington disease, a progressive brain disorder.

One of 23 Chromosomes, a single gene defect in the chromosome 4 genetic code causes steady brain deterioration known as Huntington disease[74].

Huntington's disease[75]

Science has not uncovered the purpose of the Huntington protein, nor why a few dozen repeats cause Huntington's disease.

Protein plays a central role in most diseases that lead to dementia, but researchers have not figured out what the precise role is, why the HD-related protein forms, or why the mutations are fatal.

Knowing the responsible chromosome and gene defect causing Huntington's provides hope researchers will discover a cure.

A child of somebody with Huntington's has a 50% chance of getting the disease.

V. BONUS SECTION

Whether diagnosed with dementia or preparing for a rainy day, there are basics everybody should consider.

This section focuses on steps dementia patients (all adults) should address, including forming a care team and understanding various therapy.

While written for dementia patients, I recommend every adult fulfill these tasks before you turn thirty. Waiting is our enemy for these two duties. Be prepared!

The section includes:

1. A starter to-do list for any adult diagnosed with a fatal disease such as dementia.
2. A care team plan.

Chapter 10: Starter To-do List for Somebody and Family once Diagnosed with Dementia.

Dementia patients, loved ones, and family must address several matters early in the disease, including care, financial decisions, living quarters, Living Will, and Power of Attorney.

While you have full or most of your cognitive skills, take care of the listed priorities before diagnosis or when diagnosed. Please do not consider the items covered in this section a complete care list, but a start you tailor to your needs.

Fail to cross these items off the list while you maintain your facilities causes much regret for patients and loved ones.

Your life is your ship, and for now, you remain the captain. Plan how your ship faces the coming storm and, when you can no longer captain the ship yourself, have it already determined who takes over the helm.

Now remains your last best chance to have a substantial say in your future.

Care

Family, loved ones, and dementia patients must make difficult decisions concerning if somebody can become the primary volunteer caregiver. While dementia patients do not require 24/7 care in the early stage, it becomes necessary in the middle to late stages.

Nobody can get through dementia without others providing years of caregiving. While rare dementias kill in months, most dementia patients live for 5-20 years, with dementia growing progressively worse.

Diagnosed with dementia or in perfect health, we all must ask ourselves who would take care of us if dementia or another devastating disorder struck, requiring long-term caregiving.

Most families cannot afford professional caregiving, and the government will not help until towards the end, so family and loved ones must.

In an ideal world, we ask ourselves these tough questions and have a plan in place should something happen. This benefits not only those diagnosed with dementia but also the heroic voluntary caregivers who will see them to the end.

Financial Decisions

There are significant financial decisions to make, and earlier, the better.

Find out how much your insurance covers and the amount you must pay. A kinder world would not burden dementia patients, nor their loved ones, with overwhelming medical care costs.

In the United States and most countries in the world, the majority of dementia costs fall on families.

How Much Does Dementia Cost the Average Family?

With no urine or blood test for most dementia types, neurologists must rely on imaging and other expensive tests, often not to diagnose dementia but to rule out other neurological disorders.

Under the best scenario, related tests, doctor visits saddle the average patient with tens of thousands of dollars in deductibles by the time the neurological team diagnoses them with dementia. For some, such as dementia with Lewy bodies, it might run much higher as it can take up to eighteen months or longer before doctors make a correct diagnosis.

Our health system tells the average person: "Sorry, you have dementia. Oh, by the way, there's the bill."

Doctors, medical professionals, hospitals, drug companies, and others involved in treating dementia must make a living. Even when we factor out overcharging and profiteering, treating dementia would remain expensive.

The average American family's health insurance has deteriorated for years, the premiums growing too high, the deductibles unaffordable, and too many not worth the paper its written, much less the monthly premiums.

Authorities estimate the average cost per dementia patient is $341,840, with families expected to cover 70 percent.

Such a disease becomes a hardship for not only the patient but also their family. The demands, financial and otherwise, on voluntary caregivers often is devastating. Make difficult financial decisions early.

Financial costs vary from one dementia to another and the treatment plan.

Living Quarters

While most dementia patients maintain independence in stage one, at some point, they require help with daily tasks. Will somebody move in with her or him? Does the patient move in with somebody else? Will it become necessary for him or her to move into an assisted living community in later stages? If so, what type?

The person diagnosed should gather loved ones and decide such matters in the beginning. Like somebody on a small island with a hurricane approaching, one must be diligent. While no man or woman can withstand such a storm, they still take precautions to protect themselves and their families.

In part because of financial considerations, most families care for the loved one in the home until symptoms grow critical. Whether a dementia patient ends up in a special need living facility is not a matter of if, but at what point for those who have access.

No matter how much love, care, and attention a voluntary caregiver or loved ones provide a dementia patient, they are ill-equipped to provide for somebody in the disorder's final stretch.

Families without access do the best they can to provide comfort for the loved one but make no mistake, the patient and family benefit if a special needs facility takes over at some point.

Which type of facility depends on which dementia and symptoms. Some dementias cause more cognitive problems, while others greater affect motor skills, some visual, and a few dementias cause more language problems. In the end, many dementias are more alike than not, as the damage to the brain spreads to other areas. Still, depending on the symptoms, different care facilities might be better than others.

Ask your neurologist or local dementia organizations about local facilities trained for your particular type. Hopefully, you live at home and maintain a normal or semi-normal life for years, but have a facility selected when the end grows near.

Living Will

Not to be confused with a Last Will and Testament that distributes assets, a living will focus on medical decisions. NOLO defines a living will.

> *A living will – sometimes called a health care declaration -- is a document in which you describe the kind of health care you want to receive if you are incapacitated and cannot speak for yourself. It is often paired with a power of attorney for health care, in which you name an agent to make health care decisions on your behalf. Some states combine these two documents into one document called an 'advanced directive.'*

It is crucial to document the dementia patient's wishes while you maintain facilities to make such decisions.

Use the Living Will to direct physicians to follow your wishes on what care you receive now and, in the future when you might not maintain your cognitive skills.

Specify end-of-life medical treatment.

NOLO recommends prioritizing life-prolonging medical care, food, and water if you become unconscious, and palliative care, which we soon address[76].

Distribute copies of your living will to loved ones, doctors, insurance providers, and all health care facilities.

Power of Attorney

The American Bar Association describes a power of attorney:

> *A power of attorney gives one or more persons the power to act on your behalf as your agent. The power may be limited to a particular activity, such as closing the sale of your home or be general in its application. The power may give temporary or permanent authority to act on your behalf. The power may take effect immediately, or only upon the occurrence of a future event, usually a determination that you are unable to act for yourself due to mental or physical disability. The latter is called a "springing" power of attorney. A power of attorney may be revoked, but most states require written notice of revocation to the person named to act for you[77].*

It is important to establish a medical power of attorney to empower a trusted loved one to make medical decisions when a patient becomes incapable. If you do not choose the right person, you can almost count on the wrong people making important decisions down the road.

If you're in early stages dementia and reading this, you likely can still think clearly, but this changes as the symptoms worsen. The only way to protect a dementia patient's wishes when they lose their cognitive decision making is by naming a power of attorney in advance.

Once you name a power of attorney, cover some dos and don'ts. After all, you are trusting another person with your life. Like with your doctors, speak your mind while you can and let people know what you expect.

As NOLO pointed out, some states merge the living will and power of attorney into an advanced directive. Whether together or separate, I recommend all adults, and particularly those diagnosed with dementia draw up a medical living will and name a power of attorney.

The starter to-do list provides a starting point for dementia patients, families, and any adult.

Once diagnosed, both the person diagnosed and loved ones must unite and build your to-do list. Add whatever makes sense for you and your unique situation.

Let's next cover a few key members of a dementia care team.

Chapter 12: CARE TEAM

The National Institute on Aging recommends building a care team.

The team includes an art therapist, mental health counselor, occupational therapist, palliative care specialist, physical therapist, and a speech therapist[78].

Art therapist

The art therapist reduces stress by engaging the patient in music and other expressive arts.

Since dementia causes enormous anxiety and mood swings, art therapists use music and art to soothe patients and assist caregivers. Most everybody responds to music. Some pump our blood and makes us want to shake our bodies to the rhythm. Other music helps us focus and achieve maximum concentration.

Some music geared towards dementia patients relaxes and calms. Music is a godsend!

Art is not a task but a love affair. Some say within each of us is an artist starving to escape. Art therapists use music and art as a brilliant tool to treat dementia anxiety, attention decline, sleep problems, etc.

Mental health counselors

A neurological disorder, dementia attacks the brain and inhibits cognitive skills. Mental health counselors help patients and families plan for the future and cope with the shock, hurt, and pain resulting from the diagnosis.

Most individuals and families suffer chronic mental stress when doctors diagnose a member with dementia.

Find a mental health counselor trained in dementia.

Turn to their expertise and do not allow the neurological

disorder to destroy the remaining quality of life for the patient, or respond as a family in a way where dementia destroys many lives by one sweeping event.

Occupational therapists

The occupational therapist helps patients bathe, dress, eat, and perform daily tasks.

We think of the routine daily tasks as second nature, and it is as long as the neurons, pathways, arteries, heart, and brain perform as normal. When suffering a stroke or neurological disorder like dementia, we quickly learn nothing is second nature anymore. Like a child, dementia patients often must relearn how to perform basic tasks.

Occupational therapists help patients remain independent and then semi-independent, as long as possible, extending the quality of life. An occupational therapist is instrumental in treating most dementias.

Palliative care specialist

The palliative care specialist minimizes symptoms from diagnosis to the end. You or a loved one need somebody who addresses symptoms as soon as they arise, so find a quality palliative care specialist.

They extend the quality of life and reduce suffering.

Physical therapists

Physical therapists help motors skills by leading patients through exercise.

Although dementia is known as a mental disorder, what affects the brain affects the body and vice versa. Find a physical therapist trained to work with your specific dementia.

If you've seen somebody suffering Parkinsonism or other neurological disorders affecting movement, you have an idea of the problems some dementias cause, even in the earliest stages.

A physical therapist helps maintain balance and strength, allowing a person to walk and move on their own. As dementia progresses, so does the physical therapist's importance.

Speech therapists

The speech therapist addresses speech and swallowing problems, issues present in early dementia symptoms for some types, and eventually becomes a problem for most dementias.

What is the value of verbalizing one's thoughts, understanding what a loved one says, and swallowing our food without choking or causing infection by sending it down the wrong pipe?

These are issues speech therapists excel. The ones I've observed are passionate about helping people retrain the mind to overcome aphasia and swallowing problems.

Find a speech (and other types of) therapist trained in treating your specific type of dementia. These different listed therapists can minimize the long nightmare following a dementia diagnosis.

Chapter 13: LETTER TO CONGRESS

DEAR U.S. CONGRESS, NATIONS OF THE WORLD, & WEALTHY HUMANS

We call on the United States and the governments of the world to spend less on war and walls and more on Alzheimer's and dementia research.

If aliens were attacking us from another planet, I presume the nations of the world would unite against a common enemy. That is what I propose now.

The enemy I refer to does not come from another planet but threatens humans no less. Alzheimer's and dementia strike an American every 68 seconds and somebody worldwide every 30 seconds.

The nations of the world can save millions of lives and billions of dollars.

We need necessary funding to:

1. Discover the exact cause (s) of Alzheimer's and other dementias.
2. Develop accurate testing for Alzheimer's and other dementias.
3. Develop a vaccine to wipe out Alzheimer's and other dementias like we did polio.

Alzheimer's and dementia grow at a rate that will destroy the economies of most countries if we do not become more proactive.

We can save trillions of dollars for future generations if we invest now in discovering the exact cause (s), a vaccine to prevent it from happening, and other steps to defeat this horrifying disease.

Alzheimer's and other dementias threaten every family in all nations.

We can do little for those with late-stage dementia, but the proposed steps might save millions of lives and trillions of dollars by diagnosing the different dementias early and treating them before they do significant damage.

Beller Health calls on politicians, corporations, and wealthy individuals to step forward to help win the war against dementia.

CONCLUSION

Thank you for reading this book. We covered a good amount of material.

Dementia is a cruel neurological disorder that robs people of their personalities, executive skills, memories, talents, language, voice, motor capabilities, and all that makes us individual humans.

Alzheimer's and Dementia

Although Alzheimer's disease (AD) is the most prevalent, we learned AD is to dementia what China is to Asia. Alzheimer's represents 60-80% of dementia, but 19 dementia types account for 99 percent.

Dementia Spares No Demographic

Dementia's reputation is known as an old folk's disease but strikes people all ages. Most dementia is not genetic, although certain types such as Huntington's disease are 100% familial.

Most Dementia is Incurable

Most dementia is incurable, but—if caught early enough—neurosurgeons can treat and sometimes reverse normal pressure hydrocephalus.

Dementia Prevalence

The first section focused on dementia as a general category. We learned 850,000 people in the UK have dementia, compared to 5.8 Americans and 50 million people worldwide.

Dementia Categories

We divided the 19 dementias into six categories:

- Lewy Body/Parkinsonism related dementias
- Alzheimer's related dementias
- Frontotemporal lobar degeneration related dementias
- Primary progressive aphasia related dementias
- Vascular dementias
- Other dementias

19 Dementia Types

Lewy Body/Parkinsonism Related Dementias

1. *Dementia with Lewy Bodies*
2. *Parkinson's Disease Dementia*
3. Corticobasal Syndrome

Alzheimer's Related Dementias

4. Typical Alzheimer's Disease
5. *Posterior Cortical Atrophy*
6. *Down Syndrome with Alzheimer's*
7. *Limbic-predominant Age-related TDP-43 Encephalopathy (LATE)*
8. Early-onset Alzheimer's

Frontotemporal Lobar Degeneration Related Dementias

9. *Behavioral Variant Frontotemporal Dementia*

10. _Progressive Supranuclear Palsy_

Primary Progressive Aphasia Related Dementias

11. _Nonfluent Primary Progressive Aphasia (nfvPPA)_
12. Logopenic Progressive Aphasia (LPA)

Vascular Dementia

13. _Cortical Vascular Dementia_
14. _Binswanger Disease_

Other Dementias

15. _Normal Pressure Hydrocephalus_
16. _Huntington's Disease_
17. _Korsakoff Syndrome_
18. _Creutzfeldt-Jakob Disease_
19. Amyotrophic Lateral Sclerosis

We examined Huntington's disease, defining and exploring causes, prevalence, symptoms, and stages.

THE END

Of

HUNTINGTON'S DISEASE

Continue to view other books and more information about Jerry Beller and the Beller Health Research Institute.

THANK YOU FOR READING

Thank you for reading the entire book. While this is not a literary work to enjoy, I hope you gained useful dementia knowledge.

If you benefitted from this book, please take a moment to share your thoughts in a review. Reader reviews help other readers make educated decisions about this book before purchasing.

HUNTINGTON'S DISEASE

or

https://www.amazon.com/dp/B07XLM87HL

Look for annual updates to my health books, as I follow new studies and add any helpful information I find. Health and fitness are top priorities, and the heart and brain are my specialties.

I hope you develop the habits suggested in this book. Good luck on your health journey. Live long and prosper, my friend.

All the best,
Jerry Beller & Beller Health

BELLER HEALTH BOOKS

Beller Health Research Institute specializes in the heart and brain, and published the following Jerry Beller book series:

- Arrhythmia Series
- Vascular Disease Series
- 2020 Dementia Overview Series
- 19 Dementia Types Series

Please continue to view the books in each series.

Dementia Types, Symptoms, Stages, & Risk Factors Series

This book series is the first to cover each of the 19 primary dementia types.

20. *Dementia with Lewy Bodies*
21. *Parkinson's Disease Dementia*
22. Corticobasal Syndrome
23. Typical Alzheimer's Disease
24. *Posterior Cortical Atrophy*
25. *Down Syndrome with Alzheimer's*
26. *Limbic-predominant Age-related TDP-43 Encephalopathy (LATE)*
27. Early-onset Alzheimer's
28. *Behavioral Variant Frontotemporal Dementia*
29. Progressive Supranuclear Palsy
30. *Nonfluent Primary Progressive Aphasia*
31. Logopenic Progressive Aphasia
32. *Cortical Vascular Dementia*
33. *Binswanger Disease*
34. *Normal Pressure Hydrocephalus*
35. *Huntington's Disease*
36. *Korsakoff Syndrome*
37. *Creutzfeldt-Jakob Disease*
38. Amyotrophic Lateral Sclerosis

2020 Dementia Overview Series

Whereas in the *Dementia Types, Symptoms, Stages, and Risk Factors* series, each book covers a different dementia type, this series focuses on groups of dementias.

1. Dementia Types, Symptoms, & Stages
2. *Lewy Body/Parkinsonism Dementias*
3. *Vascular Dementia*
4. *Frontotemporal Dementia (FTD)*
5. Alzheimer's Related Dementias
6. *Prevent or Slow Dementia*

Other Beller Health Books

You can view or purchase all Beller Health Books on Amazon at the following web address:

https://amzn.to/2TpDr8e

ABOUT THE AUTHOR

Jerry Beller is the lead author and researcher at Beller Medical Research Institute. Beller distinguished himself three times in the medical world by being the first to write and publish books on particular dementia fields.

He wrote the first book covering all 15 primary dementia types, which he since expanded to cover nineteen. Beller followed this accomplishment by writing a book on each dementia type. He broke medical ground a third time when he published the first book on the new dementia category LATE.

When the world struggled to grasp the difference between Alzheimer's disease and China, Beller explained:

Alzheimer's is only one dementia, much like China is only one country in Asia. Just as we do not want to ignore the other countries in Asia because China is the largest, nor do we want to ignore the less prevalent dementia types.

Despite his accomplishments, he remains humble. "Until we win the dementia war, I've no reason to celebrate," Beller said. "If we win the war during my lifetime, I will celebrate with a few hundred brothers and sisters around the world who share my passion. Until then, we have too much work left to worry about accolades and legacies."

When not researching dementia, Jerry enjoys life with his

wife of thirty-plus years, Nicola, and their two children.
Visit Jerry Beller:
https://bellerhealth.com

1 'What Is Dementia?', Alzheimer's Disease and Dementia <https://alz.org/alzheimers-dementia/what-is-dementia> [accessed 18 September 2019].

2 'What Is Dementia? Symptoms, Types, and Diagnosis', National Institute on Aging <https://www.nia.nih.gov/health/what-dementia-symptoms-types-and-diagnosis> [accessed 18 September 2019].

3 'What Is Dementia?', Alzheimer's Society <https://www.alzheimers.org.uk/about-dementia/types-dementia/what-dementia> [accessed 18 September 2019].

4 'Dementia' <https://www.who.int/news-room/fact-sheets/detail/dementia> [accessed 18 September 2019].

5 'Risk Factors' <https://stanfordhealthcare.org/medical-conditions/brain-and-nerves/dementia/risk-factors.html> [accessed 20 September 2019].

6 W. M. van der Flier and P. Scheltens, 'Epidemiology and Risk Factors of Dementia', Journal of Neurology, Neurosurgery & Psychiatry, 76.suppl 5 (2005), v2–7 <https://doi.org/10.1136/jnnp.2005.082867>.

7 Kent Allen, 'Dementia Rates to Grow for African Americans, Hispanics', AARP <http://www.aarp.org/health/dementia/info-2018/dementia-alzheimer-cases-grow-nonwhites.html> [accessed 20 September 2019].

8 Elizabeth Rose Mayeda and others, 'Inequalities in Dementia Incidence between Six Racial and Ethnic Groups over 14 Years', Alzheimer's & Dementia: The Journal of the Alzheimer's Association, 12.3 (2016), 216–24 <https://doi.org/10.1016/j.jalz.2015.12.007>.

9 'African Americans at Higher Dementia Risk than Other Racial Groups', Reuters, 10 March 2016 <https://www.reuters.com/article/us-health-dementia-race-u-s-idUSKCN0WC2X5> [accessed 20 September 2019].

10 Steve Ford, 'Likelihood of Dementia "Higher among Black Ethnic Groups"', Nursing Times, 2018 <https://www.nursingtimes.net/news/research-and-innovation/likelihood-of-dementia-higher-among-black-ethnic-groups-08-08-2018/> [accessed 21 September 2019].

11 'Dementia' <https://www.who.int/news-room/fact-sheets/detail/dementia> [accessed 21 September 2019].

12 'Women and Alzheimer's', Alzheimer's Disease and Dementia

<https://alz.org/alzheimers-dementia/what-is-alzheimers/women-and-alzheimers> [accessed 21 September 2019].

[13] 'Dementia Facts', *Dementia Consortium*
<https://www.dementiaconsortium.org/dementia-facts/> [accessed 21 September 2019].

[14] 'Dementia' <https://www.who.int/news-room/fact-sheets/detail/dementia> [accessed 21 September 2019].

[15] 'Why Is Dementia Different for Women?', *Alzheimer's Society*
<https://www.alzheimers.org.uk/blog/why-dementia-different-women> [accessed 21 September 2019].

[16] Jessica L. Podcasy and C. Neill Epperson, 'Considering Sex and Gender in Alzheimer Disease and Other Dementias', *Dialogues in Clinical Neuroscience*, 18.4 (2016), 437–46
<https://www.ncbi.nlm.nih.gov/pmc/articles/PMC5286729/> [accessed 21 September 2019].

[17] 'WHO | Life Expectancy', *WHO*
<http://www.who.int/gho/mortality_burden_disease/life_tables/situation_trends_text/en/> [accessed 21 September 2019].

[18] 'Products - Data Briefs - Number 328 - November 2018', 2019
<https://www.cdc.gov/nchs/products/databriefs/db328.htm> [accessed 21 September 2019].

[19] Jacqui Thornton, 'WHO Report Shows That Women Outlive Men Worldwide', *BMJ*, 365 (2019), l1631 <https://doi.org/10.1136/bmj.l1631>.

[20] 'Why Do Women Live Longer Than Men?', *Time*
<https://time.com/5538099/why-do-women-live-longer-than-men/> [accessed 21 September 2019].

[21] 'Dementia' <https://www.who.int/news-room/fact-sheets/detail/dementia> [accessed 20 September 2019].

[22] 'Alzheimer's Disease: Facts & Figures', *BrightFocus Foundation*, 2015
<https://www.brightfocus.org/alzheimers/article/alzheimers-disease-facts-figures> [accessed 4 September 2019].

[23] 'Facts for the Media', *Alzheimer's Society*
<https://www.alzheimers.org.uk/about-us/news-and-media/facts-media> [accessed 20 September 2019].

[24] 'Countries With The Highest Rates Of Deaths From Dementia', *WorldAtlas* <https://www.worldatlas.com/articles/countries-with-the-highest-rates-of-deaths-from-dementia.html> [accessed 20 September 2019].

[25] 'World Alzheimer Report 2018 - The State of the Art of Dementia Research: New Frontiers', *NEW FRONTIERS*, 48.

[26] 'ALZHEIMERS/DEMENTIA DEATH RATE BY COUNTRY', *World Life Expectancy* <https://www.worldlifeexpectancy.com/cause-of-death/alzheimers-dementia/by-country/> [accessed 24 September 2019].

[27] 'Alzheimer Europe - Research - European Collaboration on Dementia - Cost of Dementia - Regional/National Cost of Illness Estimates' <https://www.alzheimer-europe.org/Research/European-Collaboration-on-Dementia/Cost-of-dementia/Regional-National-cost-of-illness-estimates> [accessed 26 September 2019].

[28] 'Publications | NATSEM' <https://www.natsem.canberra.edu.au/publications/?publication=economic-cost-of-dementia-in-australia-2016-2056> [accessed 22 September 2019].

[29] 'Dementia UK Report', *Alzheimer's Society* <https://www.alzheimers.org.uk/about-us/policy-and-influencing/dementia-uk-report> [accessed 22 September 2019].

[30] 'Dementia Statistics – U.S. & Worldwide Stats', *BrainTest*, 2015 <https://braintest.com/dementia-stats-u-s-worldwide/> [accessed 23 September 2019].

[31] 'Newsroom | Northwestern Mutual - 2018 C.A.R.E. Study', *Newsroom | Northwestern Mutual* <https://news.northwesternmutual.com/2018-care-study> [accessed 22 September 2019].

[32] 'ALZHEIMERS/DEMENTIA DEATH RATE BY COUNTRY'.

[33] 'Alzheimer Europe - Research - European Collaboration on Dementia - Cost of Dementia - Regional/National Cost of Illness Estimates'.

[34] 'Publications | NATSEM'.

[35] 'Dementia UK Report'.

[36] 'Dementia Statistics – U.S. & Worldwide Stats'.

[37] 'Genetics Basics Lesson 3: Modes of Inheritance'

<http://hihg.med.miami.edu/code/http/modules/education/Design/Print.asp?CourseNum=1&LessonNum=3> [accessed 18 March 2019].

[38] Genetics Home Reference, 'Huntington Disease', *Genetics Home Reference* <https://ghr.nlm.nih.gov/condition/huntington-disease> [accessed 12 January 2019].

[39] 'Akinetic–Rigid Syndromes - Oxford Medicine' <http://oxfordmedicine.com/view/10.1093/med/9780192619112.001.0001/med-9780192619112-section-003> [accessed 30 January 2019].

[40] 'Trinucleotide Repeat Disorders', *HOPES Huntington's Disease Information*, 2010 <http://web.stanford.edu/group/hopes/cgi-bin/hopes_test/trinucleotide-repeat-disorders/> [accessed 30 January 2019].

[41] 'UPMC - Department of Pathology - University of Pittsburgh' <https://path.upmc.edu/index.html> [accessed 19 March 2019].

[42] 'Huntington's Disease', *Alzheimer's Disease and Dementia* <https://alz.org/alzheimers-dementia/what-is-dementia/types-of-dementia/huntington-s-disease> [accessed 12 January 2019].

[43] 'Juvenile Huntington Disease | Genetic and Rare Diseases Information Center (GARD) - an NCATS Program' <https://rarediseases.info.nih.gov/diseases/10510/juvenile-huntington-disease> [accessed 19 March 2019].

[44] 'Juvenile Onset HD |' <https://hdsa.org/living-with-hd/juvenile-onset-hd/> [accessed 19 March 2019].

[45] 'What Is HD? |' <https://hdsa.org/what-is-hd/> [accessed 12 January 2019].

[46] 'Population Genetics and Huntington's Disease', *HOPES Huntington's Disease Information*, 2010 <http://web.stanford.edu/group/hopes/cgi-bin/hopes_test/population-genetics-and-hd/> [accessed 12 January 2019].

[47] Victoria Divino and others, 'The Direct Medical Costs of Huntington's Disease by Stage. A Retrospective Commercial and Medicaid Claims Data Analysis', *Journal of Medical Economics*, 16.8 (2013), 1043–50 <https://doi.org/10.3111/13696998.2013.818545>.

[48] 'Early Warning Signs Of Huntington's Disease: Metabolic Changes Ahead Of Symptoms May Lead Scientists To Treatment',

Medical Daily, 2017 <http://www.medicaldaily.com/early-warning-signs-huntingtons-disease-metabolic-changes-ahead-symptoms-may-412404> [accessed 24 February 2018].

[49] 'Huntington's Disease | Memory and Aging Center' <https://memory.ucsf.edu/huntington-disease> [accessed 24 February 2018].

[50] 'Symptoms of HD | Huntington's Disease Association' <https://www.hda.org.uk/huntingtons-disease/what-is-huntingtons-disease/symptoms-of-huntingtons-disease> [accessed 24 February 2018].

[51] 'Huntington's Disease', *Nhs.Uk* <https://www.nhs.uk/conditions/huntingdons-disease/> [accessed 24 February 2018].

[52] 'Understanding Huntington's Disease', *HealthPrep* <https://healthprep.com/conditions/understanding-huntingtons-disease/> [accessed 25 February 2018].

[53] 'What Is Huntington Disease? Symptoms, Signs, Causes & Treatment', *EMedicineHealth* <https://www.emedicinehealth.com/dementia_overview/article_em.htm> [accessed 24 February 2018].

[54] Shiraz Tyebji and Anthony J. Hannan, 'Synaptopathic Mechanisms of Neurodegeneration and Dementia: Insights from Huntington's Disease', *Progress in Neurobiology*, 153 (2017), 18–45 <https://doi.org/10.1016/j.pneurobio.2017.03.008>.

[55] 'Dementia Due to Huntington Disease', *DoveMed* <http://www.dovemed.com/diseases-conditions/dementia-due-to-huntington-disease-hd/> [accessed 24 February 2018].

[56] 'Huntington's Disease - Symptoms and Causes', *Mayo Clinic* <http://www.mayoclinic.org/diseases-conditions/huntingtons-disease/symptoms-causes/syc-20356117> [accessed 24 February 2018].

[57] 'Huntington's Disease: Symptoms, Causes, and Treatment', *Medical News Today* <https://www.medicalnewstoday.com/articles/159552.php>

[accessed 24 February 2018].

[58] 'Huntington's Disease', *Your.MD*
<https://www.your.md/condition/huntingtons-disease/> [accessed 25 February 2018].

[59] '6 Early Warning Signs of Huntington's Disease'
<http://www.activebeat.com/your-health/6-early-warning-signs-of-huntingtons-disease/> [accessed 24 February 2018].

[60] 'Huntington's Disease: Symptoms, Stages & 5 Natural Treatments', *David Avocado Wolfe*, 2017
<https://www.davidwolfe.com/huntingtons-disease/> [accessed 25 February 2018].

[61] Erika Driver-Dunckley and John N. Caviness, 'CHAPTER 67 - HUNTINGTON'S DISEASE', in *Neurology and Clinical Neuroscience*, ed. by Anthony H. V. Schapira and others (Philadelphia: Mosby, 2007), pp. 879–85
<https://doi.org/10.1016/B978-0-323-03354-1.50071-7>.

[62] Celia Stewart, 'Dysphagia Symptoms and Treatment in Huntington's Disease: Review', *SIG 13 Perspectives on Swallowing and Swallowing Disorders (Dysphagia)*, 21.4 (2012), 126–34
<https://doi.org/10.1044/sasd21.4.126>.

[63] 'Huntington's Disease: Symptoms, Treatment', *WebMD*
<https://www.webmd.com/brain/hungtingtons-disease-causes-symptoms-treatment> [accessed 24 February 2018].

[64] 'Psychiatric Disorders Raise Risk of Suicidal Behavior in HD Trial Patients', *Huntington's Disease News*, 2019
<https://huntingtonsdiseasenews.com/2019/03/28/active-psychiatric-disorders-increase-risk-of-suicidal-behaviors-in-hd-trial-patients/> [accessed 4 January 2020].

[65] 'Suicide Prevention | Huntington's Disease Society of America'
<https://hdsa.org/find-help/clinical-care-services/suicide-prevention/> [accessed 4 January 2020].

[66] Jarem Sawatsky, *Dancing with Elephants: Mindfulness Training For Those Living With Dementia, Chronic Illness or an Aging Brain* (Red Canoe Press, 2017).

[67] 'Multivariate Prediction of Motor Diagnosis in Huntington's Disease: 12 Years of PREDICT-HD - Long - 2015 - Movement Disorders - Wiley Online Library' <https://onlinelibrary.wiley.com/doi/full/10.1002/mds.26364> [accessed 13 January 2019].

[68] Saul Martínez-Horta and others, 'Impaired Face-like Object Recognition in Premanifest Huntington's Disease', *Cortex*, 123 (2020), 162–72 <https://doi.org/10.1016/j.cortex.2019.10.015>.

[69] 'HD Reach□: Learn About Huntington's Disease□: Stages of HD' <http://www.hdreach.org/learn/stages.html> [accessed 13 January 2019].

[70] 'PhysiciansGuide_3rd-Edition.Pdf' <http://hdsa.org/wp-content/uploads/2015/03/PhysiciansGuide_3rd-Edition.pdf> [accessed 13 January 2019].

[71] 'Stages of Huntington's Disease', *HOPES Huntington's Disease Information*, 2011 <http://web.stanford.edu/group/hopes/cgi-bin/hopes_test/stages-of-huntingtons-disease/> [accessed 13 January 2019].

[72] 'Huntington's Disease', *Neurology* <http://columbianeurology.org/neurology/staywell/document.php> [accessed 13 January 2019].

[73] 'Stages of Huntington's Disease', *HOPES Huntington's Disease Information*, 2011 <http://web.stanford.edu/group/hopes/cgi-bin/hopes_test/stages-of-huntingtons-disease/> [accessed 13 January 2019].

[74] 'Huntington's Disease', *NORD (National Organization for Rare Disorders)* <https://rarediseases.org/rare-diseases/huntingtons-disease/> [accessed 12 January 2019].

[75] 'Huntington's_disease_(5880985560).Jpg (750×457)' <https://upload.wikimedia.org/wikipedia/commons/d/d5/Huntington%27s_disease_%285880985560%29.jpg> [accessed 12 January 2019].

[76] Betsy Simmons Hannibal and Attorney, 'How to Write a Living Will', *Www.Nolo.Com* <https://www.nolo.com/legal-encyclopedia/how-write-living-will.html> [accessed 21 November 2019].

[77] 'Power of Attorney'

<https://www.americanbar.org/groups/real_property_trust_estate/resources/esta te_planning/power_of_attorney/> [accessed 22 November 2019].

[78] 'Treatment and Management of Lewy Body Dementia', *National Institute on Aging* <https://www.nia.nih.gov/health/treatment-and-management-lewy-body-dementia> [accessed 24 April 2019].

www.ingramcontent.com/pod-product-compliance
Lightning Source LLC
Chambersburg PA
CBHW030714220526
45463CB00005B/2035